Jeet Kune Do

The Principles of a Complete Fighter

(Jeet Kune Do Training and Fighting Strategies)

Randy James

Published By **Jackson Denver**

Randy James

*Jeet Kune Do: The Principles of a Complete Fighter
(Jeet Kune Do Training and Fighting Strategies)*

ISBN   978-1-77485-867-7

No part of this guidebook shall be reproduced in any form without permission in writing from the publisher except in the case of brief quotations embodied in critical articles or reviews.

Legal & Disclaimer

The information contained in this ebook is not designed to replace or take the place of any form of medicine or professional medical advice. The information in this ebook has been provided for educational & entertainment purposes only.

The information contained in this book has been compiled from sources deemed reliable, and it is accurate to the best of the Author's knowledge; however, the Author cannot guarantee its accuracy and validity and cannot be held liable for any errors or omissions. Changes are periodically made to this book. You must consult your doctor or get professional medical advice before using any of the suggested remedies, techniques, or information in this book.

Upon using the information contained in this book, you agree to hold harmless the Author from and against any damages, costs, and expenses, including any legal fees potentially resulting from the application of any of the information provided by this guide. This disclaimer applies to any damages or injury caused by the use and application, whether directly or indirectly, of any advice or information presented, whether for breach of contract, tort, negligence, personal injury, criminal intent, or under any other cause of action.

You agree to accept all risks of using the information presented inside this book. You need to consult a professional medical practitioner in order to ensure you are both able and healthy enough to participate in this program.

TABLE OF CONTENTS

TABLE OF CONTENTS

Chapter 1: The On-Guard Stance

In discussions about stances in Jeet Kune Do that can serve as a means of attacking and

If you want to defend the best manner, the on-guard position is always in your the forefront of your mind. It is the best way to defend.

You can take this as a positive by being half bent, which is great for fighting since your body is

Always make sure you have a strong foundation which makes it simpler for you to not just attack, but to also make

defense or counterattack, as well as the reality that this could be done with no anticipation

makes it unpredictable. It also helps you relax as it gives you the opportunity to create a quick

movement. Unpredictability and smoothness makes this stance extremely efficient.

This job is also renowned for its flexibility since it offers you the opportunity to create small

moves with speed as you get close on your opponent in sturdiness and speed.

The primary instrument in this main instrument of this stance (hand and feet) are now near your opponent. They are the striking the chance of being a winner is increased to nearly 80 percent. Even a right-handed individual like Bruce Lee

It was the left hand that was accepted as he believed that the attack was performed by your

more powerful foot and hand.

The position of your arms, head, and feet is among the important aspects to be aware of when observing this posture.

If you are speaking from a left-handed fighter's stance, your shoulder and chin must be in a straight line.

Place yourself midway while lifting your right shoulder by about one-to-two inches of space before you reach your final

lower your chin by the same length. From the position you have just made up,

The bones, muscles, and joints are placed to be in perfect alignment. When you're using this position, your bones and muscles are in perfect alignment.

In close combat the head of your body will be set perpendicularly and parallel to your chin's edge in close combat.

It is pressed to the collarbone of your neck while the opposite part of the chin gets being pushed

toward the shoulder of the lead. We rarely insert the chin's point inside the lead shoulder

Shoulder, it's only performed when you are using an unwise self-protection strategy. This can cause you to

Your neck can be bent in a strange way, causing you strain your arm and shoulder, which can cause you to strain your neck.

restricting your movement since there is no support to your straight bone's muscles.

Chapter 2: The Footwork

The fundamental instrument of Jeet Kune Do dance, the reason for that is

Combatants move around. To maximize the benefits of Jeet Kune Do as a martial art, you need to be aware of how your feet. The sole determinant of your actions; it is slow

The word "footwork" means slow combat, regardless of how skilled you are at using your hands.

The essence of fighting is movement making a move to hit a target or escaping from the target.

that is why your footwork should not cause anxiety to you. It should be quick, simple and

Strong, in contrast to the traditional horse stance, which is hard to change and slow to adjust. restricting

Your speed is crucial when fighting.

In addition being able to walk with ease will aid you in attacking and defending, as well.

You will be in a position to take on any kick or punch, due to the way you move your self

It is a challenge to learn. If you can master this skill, you'll also lessen the time you utilize your hands protect yourself or defend yourself or. You can avoid virtually every

attack and at the simultaneously launch your attack and launch your own.

Apart from deflecting and defending the ball, a skilled footwork technique can assist you to get closer to your goal.

Your opponent will be able to quickly stop your from being cornered, and even keep your strength for your

attack time. Unlike when your footwork isn't as good, you could exhaust all your energy trying to

to attack your opponent mostly but with no chance of success.

In the case of footwork, the best method to use it is to put your feet in a position that is

could cause you to go in any direction extremely rapid, and you should be aware that it

You must remain in this position should there be an attacks from all directions.

Training in POWER

In the case of power, we need to correct the idea that power to strike is only the solely

Based on strength, but it is the reverse. We could have seen individuals with smaller bodies.

taking down a very built person. This is that power does not appear to be a factor when

not from your muscles, but from the power as well as the speed and acceleration of your foot and arm. We've been told about

Bruce Lee who was around 130 pounds, defeated an opponent twice.

his size , and he dominated his size with greater speed and speed of attack more than just muscle.

Additionally, it should be noted at this point to note that, in Jeet Kune Do, your attacks are triggered by the

arms should not just be used to swing it in the direction of your body, shoulders,

feet and hips as well as arms should be joined to create a powerful attack. Also, you must be aware of

the way you punch the direction it is pointing straight in the direction of your face directly in front of your nose . it

acts as a regulator, and your punch has to originate from the middle of your body and not your shoulders in the way it appears to you.

A sluggish attack with no intention of hitting or kicks will help you win fighting, as do your arms

by punching alone will not produce enough force. Your arms must be conveyors

of your power, a channel through that you are able to attack the source of your force is your body, of force

When properly utilized. A good punch can be identified when your head is positioned so that it is in alignment

by putting your foot on the front to make an even line since the body is your backbone.

working as an alliance creating the power to attacking.

Learn to squeeze your fist to the right direction to allow you to move and, if not completed,

you might sustain injury.

Chapter 3: Speed Training

What is speed in combat? It could be the speed of the element of?

Your body is primarily hands and feet? Do we have any other major elements in the body?

good? fighter? What exactly is an effective fighter?

Let's start answering the question from here the perspective that a fighter is classified as a professional when he is able to

beat his opponent faster and more powerfully, but without showing any sweat, and simultaneously

Beware of being struck by an opponent. However, this isn't the only factor that makes

A good fighter must also possess a keen sense of direction, which is precise and flawless.

stability and the ability to discern and be able to think ahead. Some individuals already possess

Certain of these skills certain of these skills require intensive training.

All the power and the strength of your body, it will be nothing when you don't have

speed since, with it out of the way, won't be able to reach the opponent in order to make them use of speed because, without it, you will not be able to utilize

strength. Speed and power are two of the things that must be considered a

success.

One of the most effective ways of increasing your speed is to be swift and abrupt in your

motion, it's identical to throwing an overhand. Take a look at the following illustration in the event of

You snap your wrist in the most recent movement while throwing a ball, it will provide the ball with a speed

Without the snap.

BRUCE LEE and THE MARTIAL BRUCE LEE AND THE MARTIAL

Within the realm of acting and martial arts, Bruce Lee stands out however, on the 20th of July 1973.

He was snatched off the the earth by death when the age was only thirty-two.

In his career as practitioner of martial arts, he began by studying Wing Chun, taking the late Yip Man as his master was able to protect himself against the shaky life he led with his family in Hong Kong. However, it was difficult for the

the martial arts, he was able to discover himself and develop an inner drive that was later a

an artist of the future and a master in martial artist made philosophers out of him.

After many years of learning in different styles of martial He was able to develop his own martial art that is appropriate

for an person. Then, the artist renamed his concept Jeet Kune Do, meaning that it was a way

of cutting off the fist. It is a martial art. Jeet Kune Do is developed not only out of his intense training

and the vastness of martial arts. This is also due to the extent of his formal understanding of philosophy.

He was able to combine his understanding of acting and his martial arts expertise which made him famous in

films like the Big Boss, Way of the Dragon, Enter the Dragon and Fist of Fury, not to be specific.

few.

Lee's passing brought sorrow in both the realm of acting as well as the world of martial arts and

it was among the reasons for a book on his fight and the man he fought was released, Tao of Jeet Kune Do.

The art of film

Of all the incredible aspects of Bruce Lee, one of the things that is worth being mentioned is his

abilities when it comes to footwork. He considered it an absolute necessity and the basis of Jeet do.

For him, the footwork process isn't only about movement, but involves things like balance the body, endurance, power

and speed. And, in other words and speed, your footwork is the best weapon for fighting.

Bruce Lee is known to have said a line about this during his lifetime. He said, "The essence of

Fighting is the process of fighting is the art of." It is a part of Jeet Kune Do, your ability to move is the main focus of fighting

because it is through it that you can reach your goal and avoid the targets. It could help you hit

and keep you from being hit.

In his lecture of the fundamental way to achieve excellent footwork. He also spoke about that the

sharp awareness of your adversaries, ability to be active, ability to discern when you may have a greater chance of winning

or even further from your opponent, and a steady posture from the start of your battle until the end or further away from your opponent.

They are the things that need to be included in the footwork.

Technically speaking your legs and hands are useless if you don't have the opportunity to gain

A correct stance when striking, if your motion is slow, it's evident that your fight is slow.

If it's fast and well-developed, you will be able strike from any angle, delivering strong hits until

the fight comes to an end. A second thing to consider in relation to footwork is that it gets you to a certain distance before

to defend yourself and avoid attacks, you should be capable of calculating your distance, also known as the duration

For this, it is known as "the combat measure." It is important to determine when to get closer to your

opponent and when to be relative to your speed of your opponent.

In terms of your footwork, you must be able to slide into and out of any place, strike from a variety of angles

and to avoid attacking from every angle. As we can see, to be a successful fighting ace, it is largely

with your feet.

FOOTWORK A DETERMINED MOVEMENT

The most widely-held belief concerning footwork, is its effectiveness lies in the bounce

However, this is not the case because Lee insists repeatedly on your movements must be

It is purposeful to ensure that you don't just bounce around for convenience or simply because you're

Masterful athletes have done seen masters perform it. Bruce Lee is known to remain in a stance motionless until he is able to see an object.

motive to strike, after which strike, then. Your movements must all be centered around one of the two reasons.

striking to avoid or avoid getting struck or avoid being struck, nothing more, nothing less.

The secret to a successful footwork is its simplicity. By making it easy it is possible to avoid the complexities of foot

movements. Think of footwork as dance movements, executed quickly, smoothly and efficiently.

Effective and free of stress. This will put you at ease and relaxed when the time comes to strike, you will be at ease and

or defend yourself if you can do it with speed and effortlessness.

Apart from the gain previously discussed, proper exercise can increase your performance in

Kicking and punching will help you save your energy and energy expenditure by simply being

Inactive for a short period of time. The benefits of correct footwork are innumerable as it enhances

the way you position your body can increase your risk of suffering a devastating attack and reduce your chance of being injured.

Additionally in the event that we consider your footwork with regard to combat, you will benefit

tremendous speed. You are able to deliver your hits , and go before your opponent can hit back with his own.

Apart from running and hitting the footwork can be used to help structure your the skills. It can be used to build your confidence

Form type of Progressive Indirect Attack to trick your opponent into the point of disadvantage It can be used to trick your opponent into a disadvantage point.

Also, you can be able to cover the distance between yourself and your competitor.

Certain martial arts, such as that of Thai Boxing, where it "hit and be hit" There are two competitors

The two hitting each other nearly equally. In this kind of scenario there is a winner the one who

is the one with the greatest endurance to pain. However, it is not the case in Jeet Kune Do, the isn't the case You must be

If you can hit your opponent, and not give them any the chance for them to strike to return the hit, you're a

smart and skilled fighter by making you almost impenetrable by your footwork.

FOUR RUDIMENTARY FOOTWORK TYPES

There are four main kinds of footwork, whereas other types you may observe are simply

Derivations of the four types kinds we're about to talk about. The four basic types are

moving forward in a descending direction, retreating forward, flanking left, and right.

PRE-FOOTWORK- YOUR STANCE

The On-Guard Stance

Before you can perform any kind of footwork, you must first be in the On-Guard Position. It is the one to be able to

Yourself that you're ready. This is the best position because of its versatility and capacity

to keep you in the know to defend and defend in a short time. It is also the topic of discussion

About because it's simple to believe. If you find it difficult to believe that something is wrong, then it could be because something else is

It is possible that something is wrong.

In this position, you should be relaxed and be able to react quickly to any motions

the opponent. The On Guard Position can also be known as"the Anchor of Jeet"

Kune Do since all skills can be mastered by it.

It's a practical option to move back and to, and around, by doing this, you won't be able to

Overstaying the duration of a position. In the On-Guard, your strongest side is allowed to lead .

Most of the time, it's your right side. it is possible to raise your most powerful hand and let it coincide with your

the shoulder to your chin and your shoulder is placed in mid-air as it allows your left shoulder rest on your right shoulder.

about an inch or two more when you lower your chin, keeping exactly the same length. The left

Your chin should be inserted into your shoulder leading position. Likewise, your left hand must be positioned as well.

You can also have a nearby spot to protect your midsection.

After this after that, you may make use of your right hand to use it as an instrument to attack, which is why you must

You should be prepared to strike anytime you want when the right side of your shoulder lifted with care while your chin is lowered

lower to prevent the jaw or chin from being attacked. Your right knee must be bent slightly to safeguard your

Your right foot needs to be twisted around 25 degrees to allow you to be able to access your

kick option. In addition the left foot must be at a 45 degrees. Then, you can raise your foot.

your heel , causing it to your heel move forward, backwards or in any direction at any time depending on the conditions.

Once you have all of this done, that you are now ready and ready to try any type of technique that you like.

strength, stamina and the ability to move.

PROGRESSION

Pace & Slip

We are primarily discussing the distance between the two of you even though

It is not intended to be an attack tool, but it is a method of getting closer to hit.

You should be pacing forward with your right leg in front , and your left leg at the rear. The rear foot should point to the side.

You are allowed to slide up to the original place of the right-foot when you make your

forward movement should cannot exceed six inches at the front and rear foot.

If you're doing this, you should ensure the same balance of your feet's weight when you walk.

one hundred percent of your weight to the front foot, while your rear leg (left) will take fifty

percent of the weight after you've completed your stepping. If you are performing the slip and pace the weight is a

You must be able to balance your weight evenly across both legs this is the most important thing to your speed and

slip.

Thrust Pace

This is primarily used for gaining proximity to your opponent. The thrust pace is more practical.

when you are using when used with PIA in conjunction with the PIA Progressive Indirect Attack. You could miss-direct your

the opponent by holding your hand and you'll be speeding up to find an area of weakness. This is also the

the only footwork method that can be used for punching , unlike the slip and pace that

It is not possible to be able to account for instant attacks when you punch. The thrust speed is usually started after you punch, and the hand is positioned prior to your feet. In addition, your body could be moving ahead of your body.

your feet while in the middle of a fight and you'll be capable of launching a counter-attack.

Shuffle Pace

It can be described as moving and dragging but all of it comes to one thing. It is an extremely

Rapid speed. It's made in one step unlike the speed and slip, which is a mixture of two.

The primary movement, which is spinning can be done using your toes as well as the balls of your feet.

Your front foot is straight and firmly planted to the floor. It is now time pushing with your back

Leg, pulling your front leg simultaneously. There should be pressure on your feet.

particularly your back leg to be able to do this correctly. However, if you start the pace, it is important to strengthen your back leg and

A gentle note, it gets stronger with time since it confuses the eyes of the unskilled from the

incredible power and efficiency it has as you put all your strength behind this ability,

your body becomes motionless, your body moves as if it were weightless.

The Burst

This can be used to achieve extremely fast punch and kick in the forward direction as it's a second thrust

and tug movements. and tug movement. Burst was originally designed for the purpose of generating an overwhelming kick, similar to the

side-kick, and then do counter-attack. This is why footwork isn't only an opportunity to

improving your skills, also transferring the ability to execute it correctly. Kicks or punches are

Good if it is derived from the good footwork.

WITHDRAWAL

It's not just in the progression of our lives that there are various forms, but also when we withdraw. The

One of the best things to the best thing about Jeet Kune Do most appealing is the fact that these different forms of progress we've created are able to be used in the same way.

The use of time can be strategy to withdraw. That's why we'll just discuss one

Removing skills that aren't necessarily the opposite of any progression technique in order to be avoided

repetition.

THE PENDULUM PACE

This is the type of pacing that is used to avoid an attack. If you take the On-Guard position,

your front leg is your right leg, is shocked to join your back leg quickly. As you move it,

at you simultaneously push your back leg and then back. In this position, your entire body

The weight will fall the lead leg, as your back foot is barely touching the ground in the single

The reason for counterbalance.

Once this is completed after that, you will be presented with the option of whether to stay on the On-Guard or to leave it.

your current position, free your current position from attack, or attempt to take the opposite of

motion as you move your back leg back to its starting position. This makes your front leg a

tool of attack.

Pendulum Pace Pendulum Pace can be seen in the very first scene from Bruce Lee in Enter the Dragon. It is also used in the film Enter the Dragon.

It is a technique that is a technique that can be used to avoid being hit , and at simultaneously launch counter-kick strikes.

FLANKING OR SIDESTEPPING

As opposed to the two previously discussed types that involve footwork, sidestepping can be utilized to stay clear of getting

strike, berate the opponent with a move whenever the opponent is in the position to strike and create a vantage point

the best way for your attack, or counterattack. What is the best way to sidestep? Bruce Lee was

One time, it was reported once said that "sidestepping shifts the burden and rearranging the position of the feet

without affecting the equilibrium."

The principle of sidestepping is to step at the side that you want to move with the feet you wish to cross

to start and must be utilized as the leading leg for the On-Guard position. For instance to start, if you

If you wish to move to the left side, you'll begin with your left foot after you have taken the Onthe left

Guard position, with your right leg in front to the left leg. This position will be exchanged. While your back leg takes its

the location you want it to be six to 18 inches at the moment could be

Your front leg is doing exactly the same.

The same strategy should be utilized when moving to the right side and your lead foot

You will be the first one to take a step, followed by the rear of your leg. You must be able to

The thought that is in your head always be aware the fact that your balance and stability is important here.

In order to master sidestepping technique requires lots of practice, not just for those who are learning

The Jeet Kune Do. It is also for anyone who is learning a form of martial art, or another. It is possible to start by learning

striking and moving with your hands and then do it with your legs until you've got a way to

Around the area. In the words of Bruce Lee will say, "It's more effective to be able to throw five punches."

Then, 20 LOUSY ones. Also, each when you punch make sure you put all your energy into the fight."

While it might be difficult and stressful, it is not difficult to learn initially, if you are able to improve your

emotions while performing a skill especially the sidestepping. With this technique, you'll soon

See a change, then take advantage of the ability to sidestep in

fighting.

FOCUSWORK FOR PRACTITIONING

As we have stated earlier in the very first Chapter of the present book that exercise is the foundation of a successful fighter, the kind of exercise that can improve your footwork is shadowboxing. This is

as, through it you'll be able to remain calm when you move, and the best way to keep your pace and not get distracted.

Your opponent and how to make use of your abilities when you move. It will give you an understanding of

that skill could be useful or not for various situations.

It can also be a way to improve your balance when making a stand and afterwards taking a step.

Any form of attack. However, other exercises are certain to aid your neuromuscular capabilities

When it comes to dealing with your body weight as well as other things, shadowboxing is among the most pure

type of exercise that will aid in improving the footwork skills you are using.

BRUCE LEE The Standard in MARTIAL ART

There are many misconceptions about Bruce Lee, one of the most common is that he was a sexy, naive man.

Many believe that he can reach the height he achieved in martial arts because the fact that he's a bit

special. This is why, even in his time the man stated that he wasn't unique, but rather

an average person who is a regular person who trains to be more efficient. The result of his extraordinary method of

the way he fights is determined by how long and intensely the athlete trained.

The more you train the more you improve by improving your endurance, posture, body

control, timing and tactics control, timing and techniques are the most important things to be aware of in combat in the same way that they are important to note in combat.

aid in harmonising your body and provide you with more comprehension of the extent to which you have

The martial arts have been largely eliminated that is, in essence is something that can be easily dealt through footwork.

THE POWER of the Dragon

It's not news anymore it was Bruce Lee trained all the days of his existence He didn't care about whether the conditions were good or not.

walking in the car, walking or going to the movies or even the book store the bookstore, he was reported to be doing just one thing

or another one that can assist in improving his martial art. He worked so for his fitness that he could not be more fit but he was never in shape.

regardless of the circumstance he encountered no matter what the circumstance. He also believed in the firm conviction that muscles aren't

Only the things that show the power.

We are going look at ways he went about his education to allow us to combine it with our own.

to our day-to-day for our daily.

The Barbell Push

For you to begin the push of the barbell it is necessary to stand firm as you expand your feet.

shoulders wide when this is completed and you're placed, you can extend your shoulders to

Grab the barbell off the ground with your hand grip while you are standing on your feet. while standing,

when you do it, maintain your elbow close to you when you push the barbell's mass out.

without bent over. Keep this position for a several seconds before returning to your original position

Then, repeat the exercise and repeat it. You can perform three sets of between eight and twelve repetitions. Then, you can repeat it again later.

You can perform 3 sets of 8, and twelve more times using your grip on the overhand.

The aim of this exercise is to strengthen your shoulders, forearms and forearms. Biceps, forearms and biceps.

Abs, triceps, laps and chest. In reality, it could appear to be like a challenge (nothing bad comes from it).

Simple) however, it's very efficient when it is a full body workout.

Punching with a Dumbbell

It is done by holding a dumbbell between both of your hands. After that, adopt a stance of fighting; it is recommended to do this the On-Guard Stance before launching punches. Bruce Lee was known for this because he

The five-pound dumbbells in his hands while was throwing punches at the same time as he alternated

the hands.

If you are doing this workout it is important to be moderately fast in order not to cause injury to yourself. Perform this exercise

In two to three sets that take between ten and fifteen reps for each set. Do two to three sets and do ten to fifteen reps per.

One-Hand Dumbbell Drill

If you are planning to perform this exercise, you'll first need to stand up with your feet spread out in

shoulders wide while you hold using your right hand, the dumbbell of five pounds to be held shoulder-width wide. allow your shoulders to be spread out

arm, and keep it at your side while you use only your wrist to raise the dumbbell to the highest level you can.

is feasible, bring it down until it's not further.

The aim of this workout is to allow your wrist to be strong enough to punch powerful punches.

It's designed to assist you in making a powerful close-range punches, and was utilized in the case of Bruce Lee to

Improve his punch of one inch.

To ensure the efficacy of this workout Perform 2 sets of 25 reps prior to performing two sets.

sets of 25 reps while you move your wrist from one side to the next taking note of each

point break.

It is the Isometrics of Punching

This is a most popular exercises for Lee because it increases your speed and punching power.

To participate in this sport game, you will require rope. You could use a jump ropes, which are a sturdy rope

or a karate belt.

Start by putting yourself in an aggressive position. You grab the belt or rope using your hands. After that, you

place your left hand on your back while you wrap one end of your shoulder.

Finally, you'll be able to make a short-range kick. You should hold this for around five seconds, before you extend the punch up to three quarters, and you'll be on it for another five seconds , and then

Finish it off with a full-on punch while you are at the rope.

To maximize effectiveness, perform this for 5 sets with five reps , alternating the hands.

Board Isometrics

Before we begin, it is important to remember it is a meant for the leg in the way it develops.

its power and flexibility. It all starts by purchasing an eight-foot long board that is securely strapped

between the shoulder in the middle by the shoulder harness. Then, adopt a combat place on the board, as you

The harness is wrapped around your neck while you press upwards steadily while you lean toward the

Front and rear.

Even though this exercise is at the extreme side it increases the intensity of your rage and aids you

to create powerful distancing. Making three minutes of sets each is an excellent idea to begin

But it is recommended to increase the amount as time passes.

Hand Isometrics

This is a variant of the general isometrics since it's an exercise that can help you strengthen your

forearms are great to punch and trapping. Like other boards, your forearms are good for punching and trapping.

You'll need the board.

Place your feet by a shoulder-width direction as you place the harness on your forearms.

when you press upwards. Pressing upwards for three sets of one minute, with you still seated with nothing

More than a minute in between sets can be effective , but as time passes on, you'll be able to

Make it longer.

Punching with the Bull Worker

A set of two to three sets will be beneficial because you can throw back a fists, or straight punches.

One of the aspects that makes this drill unique is that it instructs the participant on how to respond and control your emotions.

the pressure that surrounds you when you fight.

Trapping using the Bull Worker

As with the previous exercise You will require to use Bull Worker, this empowers

Your forearms are ready for you to catch, grab and strike.

Make sure to keep a fight posture while you place one edge of the Bull Worker alongside your abs while you

Take the other end and place it in approximately the height of your head. Next, in a rapid motion, pull the upper

The part that is toward your part in the direction of your abs. Release before repeating this each time.

Chapter 4: Of Bruce Lee's Training Philosophy

The Tao of Jeet Kune Do will teach you the way Bruce Lee arrived at his personal truth, which he termed Jeet Kune Do (JKD). The method he followed is a simple and concise approach that every martial artist can apply to their own journey. Here's how:

Bruce Lee Training Philosophy Concept #1

SEEK the truth

You must be consciously seeking to understand the truth.

Find it. Learn about the real world of fighting by yourself. Do not rely on the advice of your instructor, former masters, or other martial artists say is true. Make your own research. You will not learn by doing your neighbor's homework.

Every opportunity is a good one to research what actually happens in an self-defense or assault scenario -- not only physically

1

But also mentally. What effect was anxiety, fear and anger affect the incident?

Bruce Lee Training Philosophy Concept #2

AFFIRMATIVELY AWARE

Be aware of what you're looking to find and don't lose your mind when you find it. Martial artists who've devoted hours of study in a traditional style and followed the rules they've been taught as the truth, sometimes find it difficult accepting that they may have been engrossed in a lie for a long time. They may not have studied a lie but they may also have trained for years according to the lie.

The most important thing is to avoid dwelling on the falsehood. You should be grateful that you've become conscious of the issue, and adapt your methods according to what you've learned is true.

Bruce Lee Training Philosophy Concept #3

Perceive the truth

Perception is everything in all aspects of life, and even in fighting arts. Create your perceptions as complete in nature as you possibly can. Find as many details as you can about the topic or the situation prior to making a decision.

Bruce Lee Training Philosophy Concept #4

Experience the truth

If you find something you believe to be factual assertion test it by putting on the examination. Most of the time, this is putting on your protective gear and making full contact in a real-life situation.

This is a vital element of finding out the truth, a task which many do not accomplish. Bruce Lee was fond of saying that you can't be a swimmer without first getting into

Bruce Lee's Training Philosophy 3

the water. You can't train to be an effective fighter without fighting.

One word of warning how to determine if the information you're trying to test is worth your time If the truth is applying a technique that you're not familiar Don't be impulsive to dismiss it in the event that it fails. We all know that it requires time and effort to understand a new skill. The technique's failure could be the result of inadequate execution, not necessarily from poor design.

Bruce Lee Training Philosophy Concept #5

MASTER THE TRUTH

When you've uncovered an untruth or experienced it, you can then

It was proven to be true discovered it to be true, learn how to master the fact. It involves repetition of drills and execution. Like you would have done during your own experience try it out from every angle against different adversaries in as many situations as you can. Include it in your regimen of training.

Bruce Lee Training Philosophy Concept #6

DO NOT FORGET THE TRUTH, AND THE CARRIERS of the TRUTH

How do you know what Bruce Lee mean by this? If what you learnt was the art of punching and the vehicle for the truth could be boxing. After you've learned your hand-hand abilities you no longer requirement to link them to boxing. It was just a means for getting you to where you needed to get to. It is a fact that belongs to the person who created it. The truth of one person could be someone else's restriction. In not being bound by the system, you can avoid these restrictions. You've absorbed what's valuable and disregarded those that are not useful.

Bruce Lee Training Philosophy Concept #7

REPOSE IN THE NEXT THING

There is no way to rest in the happiness of knowing that

The truth you've discovered is likely to change over the passing of time. A long time ago, the defense of an empty hand against a sword may be a fact however, today it's extremely unlikely to encounter someone who wields the weapon. However, a baseball bat or knife attack is entirely possible. The actuality of a sword-attack has changed, or maybe "evolved" is the better term. The reality is that what you learn today could be the story you heard yesterday is no longer the case.

If you're a student who is just beginning to learn martial arts, you must learn the various exercises and jeet kunedo techniques covered in this section prior to proceeding to the sparring section in the book or engaging in any sparring the practice room.

The exercises should feel secure and comfortable. the instructor should be cautious in feeding any technique which may cause physical contact. The instructor should begin slowly and gradually increase the speed until full speed after the student proves that he is able to manage the task. The best part about this type of instruction is that it helps both of the players. While one team member is working on defensewhile the others will take advantage of offense.

Gunfight Sciences

Gunfight!

What do you think of when you hear this?

The fictionalized representation of the image we make out of our minds when we hear "gunfight," for most people in all likelihood, stems from the stories that movies and television want us to believe.

A "gunfight" is basically the sight of two Old West gunfighters squaring off with one another on a dirt road or in futuristic close quarters fighting with guns that resemble the films that feature John Woo and Kurt Wimmer.

The overly romanticized depictions of gunfights were first introduced in dime novels in the 19th century, and continued to be popular during the film time.

In reality in reality, what was "real" gunfights in during the Old West were rarely that "civilized."

5

In reality there are many erroneous information regarding this "romanticized" gunfights The first is that, very rarely, did those involved actually "plan" to allow an actual gunfight to happen.

The other part is "calling for the "calling" of their foe for dueling in the streets. The majority of these fights were fought during the hot moments where tempers were raging, and, more often than not using the tiniest bit of dark-bottled courage.

They were also not in a radius of 15 feet in the gunfight, each participant taking only one shot, and one falling to the ground dead while the other stood as an "hero" in front of crowds of onlookers.

The fights were generally close and intimate, with a variety of shots fired by those "six shooters" and often leaving innocent spectators being hit by a bullet that escaped. In many fights, it was difficult to determine who been the one who "won" for a long time until the smoke of black powder was gone.

Like today's gunfights in a battle zone, it's typically caused by an ambush, or a raid.

Ambushs are the most frequent one, which causes our soldiers to respond by devising a counter-ambush strategy before executing the plan.

For our soldiers, it is a blessing that they've left FOB (forward operating base) adhering to two rules of gunfighting: #1 Take A Gun and #2 - Bring Friends With Guns! Modern-day firearms and the history behind them continues to be extensively studied. Many devote their entire lives to enhancing their gunfighting techniques and tactics.

In addition, they adopt their mentality in the same way that the way a Samurai Warrior committed his

Gunfight Sciences 7

mental state, allowing the mindset to influence the body's reactions and actions.

We as 2nd Amendment expressing gun carriers prepare for the possibility of a deadly shoot by continuing to drive to the range in a static position and then punch the smallest holes we can in targets made of paper.

Our ethos is that we'll be able to confront an adversary in front and triumphantly defeat him using our superior shooting skills . Then, we look at the gorgeous woman we saved and give her a smile, and ask "Are you okay?"

We have a habit of constantly working on the areas of shooting that we are naturally proficient at. The strong-handed weaver , or isosceles posture is the standard image of the man right next to you, and more likely that you too!

While it is a great starting point for a beginner but the true warrior needs to be prepared for the fight of a lifetime which will be confronted.

In order to do this, you have to get from your normal routine, and work on the things we're not experts at.

Are you prepared enough to fight a fire?

The Science Of A Gunfight

In today's gunfights in a battle zone it's typically caused by an ambush or raid. Ambush is the most frequent and causing our soldiers to respond and devise a counter-ambush plan before executing the plan. For our soldiers, they've left their FOB (forward operating base) adhering to these rules #1 and #2 of gunfighting. #1

Take A Gun and #2 - Bring Friends With Guns! Modern-day guns and the history behind them continues to be thoroughly studied. Many devote their lives to improving their gunfighting abilities and tactics. They also adopt their mentality in similar ways to the Samurai War. Samurai War

9

The rior committed his mind and allowed his mindset to influence the body's reactions and actions.

We often as 2nd Amendment expressing gun carriers prepare for our upcoming battle by continuing to visit an indoor range and make the smallest holes we can in paper targets. The idea is that we'll knowingly engage the enemy in front of us and defeat him with our exceptional shooting abilities, then look at the gorgeous woman we saved and give her a to her and say "Are you okay?" We are guilty of constantly practicing those aspects of shooting that we naturally excel at. The powerful weaver, also known as the isosceles posture is the standard image of the man who is right in front of you, and more likely also you!

While this is a good starting point for a beginner but the true warrior needs to be prepared for the fight of a lifetime that is brought to bear. In order to do this, you need to step away from the comfort zones and practice on the areas we're not able to master. Our minds must be trained to notice things that we may miss if not paying attention to them. We need to be aware of the fight space, then move into it with determination, and take over the battle.

To comprehend the fundamentals of gunfights it is necessary to broaden your knowledge a bit beyond the simple trigger pulling. When you think about modern-day gunfights or dealing with any kind of threat There are four ideas I recommend you consider. I would like you to incorporate them into your thought process to ensure that while you are studying, practicing, and even out in the open, these ideas become natural to you. When you are familiar with how to apply the Science of Gunfighting then your training, and ultimately , your fighting will be given an entirely new significance.

There is first threat vector. This is the direction of attack that the threat is following directly towards you. It doesn't matter if it's an attacker physically such as a knife or even an actual bullet, the route which is the straightest route to you is called your threat vector. It could be from any direction and not be limited to the two scenarios that you've played repeatedly in your mind. The threat vector defines the action and reaction requirements , and also helps to define the subsequent concepts.

The second is SPACE. Space is the immediate space that you need to manage with threats. To define space, begin by asking yourself these questions: What is in the vicinity? Where are you able to go? Where are they going? Are there any opportunities in the vicinity that could be used to tilt the advantage to your favor? Are you close to the danger? Utilize these questions to determine the location you are in so that you can determine the best way to avoid being in the area for the bullet to hit or the knife to cut, or for the bullet to strike.

The third idea is TIME. The duration of a gunfight specifically, is determined by the threat vector and/or space rather than the physical capacity to draw or leave the lines of attack. Consider: can I get away? Will I be able to locate my weapon at the right time to protect myself? Do I have enough time to safeguard my children or do I need to act immediately? Do you see the threat and process it, manage your response, and then take action before he had reduced the distance to the threat direction?

The final concept is FORCE. Force is the immediate threat posed by the attack. When it comes to physical attacks for example, a hand-to hand fight that involves using power against him is more effective than overcoming him. There are some issues with trying to take on one. In the effort to overwhelm your adversary, you may apply too much power , causing injuries to him that are not needed and resulting in expensive (and possibly embarrassing) legal troubles. In court, the notion to use "appropriate use of force" to deter the threat is employed. Your counterattack must be equivalent to the judge's eyes the judge, to the one the threat that you face. Remember, the criminal decides on the timing, location and amount of force to be used much like an ambush that troops confront. We're not able to predict the future "scenarios" are nothing more than thoughts of potential scenarios that may not have any connection to the reality of the present situation. This is why we prepare for everything, as absurd as it may sound It's impossible to predict the exact time or location where your situation will unfold.

In hand-to-hand combat, with your physique against an opponent gives you more options , and will require less movement and strength to fight them. It is almost always the case that this benefit keeps you fighting for longer since your fatigue is less apparent. When it comes to gunfights it's not about who shoots first, but who is the first to fire and who hits first! A precise hit can end gunfights quickly!

How do these concepts interconnect to form science?

"Science" is a reference to an entire body of knowledge which can be explained rationally and applied consistently. In 19th-century, the term "science" was increasingly connected with the scientific method as a method of discipline to learn about the natural world. This includes geology, chemistry, physics and biology. Through observations and experiments, aids us to identify the basic principles and develop theories. These expressions then are transformed into knowledge. In order to gain knowledge, we must consider how we can acquire authentic knowledge using the various kinds of learning methods.

The three most commonly used kinds are (in any order at all)

• Spatial enjoy studying through images and pictures

• Linguistics: are more comfortable using words in both speech and writing

"Kinesthetic": enjoy using your hands, your body and a sense of contact.

The majority of us learn through "doing" rather than reading, lecturing or looking at images. Kinesthetic learning is the process of learning where the student uses the movements to acquire information about the surroundings that they are living in. Utilizing movement into your training will help reinforce the ideas discussed here. In the majority of gunfighting classes, you will be taught when you detect threats to "MOVE"! Move away from the threat vector to gain more space. If we are able to practice understanding these concepts, we will naturally apply them in stressful situations. Similar to an kinesthetic student, you'll be able to identify these elements when they appear, however lacking the understanding to apply the information we have, we'll not make the right choices.

It brings us back to a different aspect of learning, Retention as opposed to. comprehension. Retention is similar to studying the night before taking a exam. We absorb all the information we can in order to be able to efficiently recite the next day, only to forget it a week or day later. The ability to comprehend is a skill we can apply repeatedly regardless of the circumstances (or the situation). Recognizing that the majority us are kinesthetic learners and getting up from our seats to begin "doing" it can lead to understanding. To put it into context and to tell you the threat that is in front of you, and then pivot your weak front foot towards the rear and draw, will bring about what you are capable of picturing and imagining within your mind. It's not a part of your memory, nor does it have the ability to be effectively applied in a"time is real" scenario when you're under duress and stress. However, if I show it to you and make you repeat it repeatedly (this could require several shooting lessons to master) until it becomes instinctual (passing the retention part of learning) You will be equipped with the skills and knowledge to execute it correctly. This is because the method of learning was used to make it more clear and that is why taking just two or three shooting classes might not be enough to prepare you for gunfights contrary to what some instructors inform you.

Ok! Let's stop talking about the professor Let's get into the form!

In all situations, detection of threat and its vector occurs first. It is then that your brain has identified the kind of threat. In the past it is impossible to know in what direction the threat is likely to take until it is able to be found, which puts us in the defensive. Moving away from the defensive means that we are reacting. When we train, for example, when we turn our backs to the danger we are training our brains to apply the skills that we acquired through kinesthetic training to be able to respond appropriately. This is a way of controlling our time and space more effectively. After both the vector and threat are determined, we can calculate the area we will need to work in. Space covers not only the your distance from the danger as well as your space of moving away of the danger. If we're at home and a window has recently damaged, we must decide what to do. This is taking up our precious time and understanding the space around us is crucial. If you've seen spy films like those of the Jason Bourne types you will frequently see our hero walking in a cafe or another kind of establishment, and taking note of the exits, entrances, and different types of obstructions. Actually, this is performed by the OGA (other federal agencies) personnel during actual missions. They're in the process of determining their "space" and also, as performing mental game of imagining possible avenues of attack.

It is possible to do this from our at home! It is possible to look at the way our bedroom, or safe space is laid out as well as the potential options for movement. It is possible to consider ways we can use this space so that we can use it towards our advantage. Are there any chests of drawers we could throw across the front door, thereby slowing his entry in the area? Are there windows to escape from? There are endless possibilities. When you hear about a house attack, the victim hides in the cupboard "hoping" for a chance to not be discovered. Perhaps this was their only option , but when we know our own space we have the best chance to fight.

The importance of time is in the timing! It is the only way that we have the ability to actually devise an action plan. We didn't create the exact time for this particular event, the king did, and we have to take it on with aplomb. Based on our perception of threats and its vector , we can decide on what we can afford to accomplish in our space. In our training, we often utilize shot timers in order to measure the overall speed and ability with a particular exercise. It can help us increase stress and force our performance to a greater performance than we believed was could be. There will not be an actual shot timer in your vicinity, but making your opponent's threat visible before he gets you will win in every book. If you're in a position to have time and the ability to leave, you can leave. If not, you should get started getting to work on what you're planning to take on!

Once you have this information you are now able to calculate the force you must apply to the vector time, space, and distance you think you can stop, deflect, or stop the danger. Remember that in a gunfight the first rule to follow is "Bring A Gun!". If you put it in your car or sat at home in the safe, it's useless. When the time comes and you are required to take the smoke-filled wagon out, you'll definitely be tempted to employ the three concepts we have that are discussed in this article. The entire process of training, or lack of, will end in a flash of an eye. The majority of people who have been engaged in gunfights report that the pace of time slowed and the whole thing seemed unreal. This is because our brains are processing the event at a greater speed than our bodies can. Training during stress can increase the possibility of executing correct actions in the right timeframe with positive results.

"Gunfighting" or the "science of fighting" takes place when these four concepts are brought along with the bodily movements that your body performs. Your brain will only instruct that your body to act if you've practiced to do it. .... Everything else is an anxiety! We hope that you are more aware of the reasons we have been so effective in engaging our adversaries abroad. The military utilizes these concepts beginning on the first day of entry. They continue to study the art of combat in order to ensure that perfection is achieved on the battlefield. The goal of a perfect gunfight is when the enemy dies to defend his cause, and you eating breakfast the following morning.

Although science is used to determine actions, knowledge helps us define the nature of our reactions in turn converting the instinct into actions. Animals are driven by instinct. They aren't aware of or comprehend why they're doing what they do the things they do. They just do. It isn't always "doing" the best choice to take. Humans have an in-depth understanding of our minds as well as our surroundings and apply this understanding to make better choices. Utilizing these knowledge, and exercising with determination will give you an advantage in the battle.

Although science can seem complicated however, it's not... an effective method of avoiding injury. most effective method of avoiding being shot, punched shot, or slashed is to be safe and not in the area!

Be careful not to stay there...move away from the direction!

Be careful not to be there...gain or eliminate space before your adversary does!

Do not be there...recognize the moment and act to the situation!

If you're there...apply the appropriate force!

...And you thought all the gun people talked about was guns!

Keep an eye on the ball and practice often!

Jeet Kune Do Warm-Up Exercises

Warm-up exercises are a vital component in Kung Fu training. The muscles in the body can be prone to injury when they're not adequately warm and limber.

Prior to each session, warm up by performing some fundamental exercises. Practice all movements slowly as well as fast, while being soft and hard. The efficacy in Jeet Kune-Do depends on split-second timing and reflexive movement that can be accomplished only by repeated training.

When you perform the moves make sure to utilize your imagination. Imagine your opponent fighting, and then use Jeet Kune-Do techniques in response to this imaginary attack.

As these methods become more inseparable, new meanings will be revealed and more effective techniques is formulated.

Students of Karate who are complaining about push-ups with knuckles could try them using two fingers instead of just one hand!

Fitness is an essential part for everyone who trains for Martial Artists. Bruce Lee doing two-finger and thumb push-ups is an exercise routine that he does every day to tone his body.

JKD Tips for Training

In order to improve your jeet kunedo methods effective, you have to be able to work against an opponent that is trying to hit you. Since this kind of training could cause injuries, you should begin slowly and gradually. It is also important to ensure that you are able to trust your trainer and that you are willing to assist each to help each other. In order to do this, you'll have to let go of your ego and accept that regardless of how skilled you may be, everyone is going to get knocked down at some point during the time they fight.

In order to make the student feel at ease with full-contact kunedo, begin by teaching him boxing safety drills. This kind of training involves blocking, learning how to roll with a punch and many other techniques that are passive. While passive techniques are best avoided when self-defense is the goal but they can be necessary.

The passive moves may come useful in real-life like during the "oh is that" moment where you're confused and don't have opportunity to accomplish anything other except hit or block. The main characteristic of passive techniques is that they allow an opponent the opportunity to launch another attack. If you hit and block you, the opponent will have the room to attack. This is why the most important element to develop in jeet kunedo is to be able to block the opponent's attacks with an end-of-hit or stop-kick.

After that, you can drill using straight lead punches. Followed by straight rear kicks, after which you can add hooks as well as other boxing punches. Always start these drills at the combat measure to give the student time to respond. After that, move forward until the instructor doesn't need to go ahead. Defense is typically required when the opponent has closed the gap. This is the reason you'll need to practice defense drills by having the trainer execute jeet kunedo moves from a distance.

Although the hand-matching drills can be performed right lead against left lead, a portion of time should be devoted to Left leads against Left leads. Similar is the case for unmatched leads as well as left-to right leads.

Regarding kicks after the student is able to kick with a bit of speed and precision then you can begin to drill defense. As with hand tools the instructor will strike with a kick or punch and the pupil will respond with the correct defense. After the student is taught the basics of defense when in a static place, the instructor uses the footwork to move and attack. Keep in mind that you're just limited to your imagination!

One of the most overlooked aspects of martial artists is physical exercise. A lot of time is spent learning the ability to master techniques but too little time is spent on physical activity. Training your skills in fighting is essential but it is equally important to maintain your physical fitness. In reality, both are required for success in combat. Training is a method that helps you discipline your mind, building your endurance and strength, and also providing strength to your body.

Aerobic Exercises

Lee's daily regimen was comprised of aerobic exercise, along with other exercises that were designed to help him improve his skills in combat. Lee varied his workouts to keep him from getting bored. One of his most favorite workouts was running four miles every day in between 24 and 25 minutes. He would alter his pace when running. After several miles of continuous or regular strides, he would sprint for several feet before he would back to running more easily. In between tempo changes as well as shuffle his feet. Lee did not care about which areas he ran at: on the beaches, in parks or woods, down and up hills, or on streets with pavement.

Apart from running, he rode an exercycle in order to build his endurance, legs , and cardiomuscles. The exercycle was usually used at in full speed, ranging from 35-40 miles per hour up to 45 minutes one hour. He would often ride his bike right after running.

Skipping Rope

Another aerobic activity that Lee included in his workout regimen was skipping rope. You can use. It not only builds your leg muscles and endurance but also enhances your performance, it makes it possible to be "light and agile." Just recently, scientists have discovered, through numerous tests that skipping rope is more effective than running. 10 minutes of skipping rope is the same as 30 minutes of running. Both are excellent exercises to strengthen the cardiovascular system.

The correct way to use rope is among the most effective exercises to develop a feeling of balance. Start by skipping on one foot while holding the other side in front of you. After that, move your foot around, jumping on the other foot for each turn of the rope, ranging from an easy pace up to a very fast speed. Limit your arm's swing, instead using your wrists, make the rope swing over. Your foot should be lifted slightly over the ground, just enough to allow the rope to go through. You should do this for 3 minutes (equivalent to a round of the boxing game) and then take a rest for one minute before continuing to do another round. 3 rounds of the workout is enough for a solid exercise. When you're accustomed to skip, you may cut out the rest and perform the exercise for up to 30 minutes in a row. The most effective rope is made from leather that has ball bearings within the handles.

Shadowboxing and Sparring

Another endurance exercise is sparring and shadowboxing. Shadowboxing is an excellent training exercise for agility that can also build your speed. Let your muscles relax and begin learning to move smoothly and effortlessly. Begin by focusing on your posture and then move easily to your feet till it feels effortless and comfortable. then, work harder and faster. It's an excellent idea to begin your exercise with the shadowbox to loosen your muscles. Imagine that your most formidable opponent is standing in front of you, and you're going to destroy him. If you can use your imagination with a lot of force, you can create your mind with a real mental battle. In addition to building stamina, shadowboxing speeds up your speed, sparks strategies and ideas that can be applied spontaneously and instinctively. Doing multiple times is the most effective method to master how to properly footwork.

A lot of beginners are just in a state of utter dozing off. Only through consistent and hard training will you build endurance. It is necessary to push yourself to exhaustion ("out out of breath" and anticipate muscle pain within a few days). The most efficient method of endurance training is a long duration of exercise, interspersed with several short, high-intensity exercises. Exercises that build stamina must be gradually and slowly increase. Six weeks of exercise is the minimum requirement for all sports that require a lot of endurance. It takes a long time to get at peak performance And unfortunately, stamina can be lost quickly in the event that you stop your high-intensity exercises. Based on the opinions of some health professionals the majority of the benefit you get from exercising in the event that you miss more than a single day between exercise sessions.

Self Defense Lessons

WARNING! Don't ever apply what I've taught unless your own life or that of your loved ones are at stake. Don't be a fighter for pride or ego. My B.E.T. System is only to be used in an emergency situation that could be life or death.

Within my B.E.T. "Target and Self Defense" Self Defense System , I instruct individuals to hit specific targets in the body of an attacker in order to trigger an emotional reaction that opens the second target to take out the threat in just a few minutes.

The movement I'm demonstrating on this clip is the Trachea (also known as a throat strike) that uses the ulna bone on my forearm.

I don't teach complex techniques that you'll forget in a life-or-death scenario.

In this video, I am simply making my body look like an attacker and then striking their trachea using the ulna bone in my forearm. I also demonstrate how to move

27 28 The Tao Of Juu Kune Do

Through the attacker, you will have your ulna bone placed in the fixed place.

In addition to striking, I will also move my body weight over the attacker to inflict further injury so that I can remove the threat as quickly as I can and then either go on towards a different menace (second attack) or leave the area. I select the trachea as an area of attack because it is the main route of air to the lungs.

If I block my attacker's breathing then they'll quickly cease to function and no longer a threat to me and my entire family (if they are in my presence during an attack).

The trachea is crushed and causes the attacker to be asphyxiated and their hands to fall into their throats. It can also make the attacker panic. The trachea can be opened by hitting it. an additional target, where I could further aggravate the injury by attacking a different victim.

The majority of gyms in the area will have this kind of equipment to use, or you can buy it online or local shop.

I prefer using a BOB since it's more realistic. You can also play with a partner, however, you must be extremely cautious and take your time moving so as to not hurt your partner in practice.

Self Defense Lessons 29

Fighting Ranges

Most people have been familiar with the four types of combat: kicking grappling, trapping, and punching. They are most likely related to training in jeet kune do, a form of martial arts in which participants attempt to learn various skills in different disciplines in order to make themselves ready to take on any challenge.

However, there's an additional range set that are just three this time during JKD training. These are the middle, high and lower ranges. If you are trained to strategically make use of them, you will make yourself a better combatant and your opponent to a fool that gets removed from the fight quicker, with less effort and more effectively.

Fight with shrewdness

Physically speaking, Bruce Lee was not a huge man. With a weight of around 130 pounds, Bruce Lee had to be sure of that his methods and strategies were effective.

These were the most efficient and realistic models that have been made. JKDconcepts ' instructor Ralph Bustamante is in the same boat. "I'm at 150 pounds currently, and this is most likely the largest I've ever measured," said Ralph Bustamante who is certified by Burton Richardson and has trained with Dan Inosanto, Richard Bustillo and the Machados. "For me to be able to do something I need to master the technique But only technique isn't going help me get to there I'd like be."

This is where the three ranges are crucial. The general strategy goes like this: When an adversary attacks you from one area, your attention is solely on that particular range. The best solution for you to counterattack your opponent in a different range.

"When someone is performing something within one area, they're not thinking about the other ranges" stated Ralph Bustamante, who teaches JKD in Santa Clarita, California. "If you're caught during a battle it's important to consider the ranges that you're not considering."

Definitions

If you are in a battle the opponent regardless of his level of trainingis able to easily target you from all three possible ranges. If you use the high range, you could see him hit you in the face. If you use the mid range, you may make a hook for your bread basket or knee towards your sternum. In the low level, he may throw a kick towards your knee or thigh.

The secret to using JKD's three ranges is safeguarding the body part of your opponent attacks with blocking, evading, or intercepting before counterattacking at an alternate area. Doesn't that sound simple, does it?

"It requires a bit of training to master these ranges" stated Ralph Bustamante who has been training in combat sports for over 30 years. "First you need someone to be able to prove that they exist. For those who have no experience, they don't realize they have the ability to fight at in a different way. They're like they've got rules that outline what they are allowed and not permitted to do in combat. However, constantly being confronted with the fact that you have alternatives and having training to ensure you know what the alternative is, can give you an edge."

Why aren't more martial artists have the knowledge to utilize the ranges? "A majority individuals have had exposure to them, but they appear to be pushing them to the other side," Ralph Bustamante said. "I believe that's because they are trying to smack heads, they are looking to compete against them on similar levels. This isn't the best approach unless you're fighting in a tournament. In the street, you'll need to be prepared to confuse and mix up your opponent. You are able to do this by attacking the various distances."
Refusal

The average martial artist aspires -- and trainsto beat his adversaries by using whatever skills he can master most well, Ralph Bustamante said. It's possible to win when your opponent is skilled at a particular range (say the boxer) but you're skilled at other things (a proficient muay Thai thigh kicker for instance.).

What happens if both the two of you both happen to be punchers of a certain level? It is possible that you will be slugging your opponent in a non-rules boxing match. However, this is typically the result of traditional training where students compete with others similar to them Boxers fight with other boxers, taekwondo instructors throw other taekwondo students or kick other taekwondo practitioners.

Afflicting an attacker with a weapon which he's never experienced and, consequently, isn't adept at protecting against, is more sensible. "I've had to deal with a few kickboxers who were skilled in their craft," Ralph Bustamante said. "But when they attempt to master the various styles, they're confused. They're surprised since it's not the range that they're used to."

If three ranges are utilized effectively, martial artists who are shocked are usually filled with disbelief. "A often it's denial" Ralph Bustamante said. "They aren't sure how to interpret it. They're eager to do it again, but usually, they fail because they're not competing at the same scale."

When it comes to an average tournament or mixed martial combat, it's fairly simple to identify your opponent's manner of fighting before you get into a battle. On the other hand how do you be sure? "You never really know what a person will do," Ralph Bustamante said. "If you're a street fighter you can grab something from the ground which will throw everything away in the sense of wanting to come over and fight with him. However, most will pounce on you and drag you down." Some will attempt to punch you on the head. The best thing you can do, Ralph Bustamante said, is to stay clear of your opponent and understand the way he fights.

Once you've determined the style of his character -- you can tell he's a hunter, for instance -- this is your signal to look for the mid or low range. "The first thing to consider is: 'What's you doing?' as whatever he's up to, you shouldn't be doing," he said.

Utilizing the jeet kunedo ranges previously mentioned doesn't require you to take on and beat your opponent by using the range you're not comfortable. It's more like that you employ a particular range to cause anxiety, and then change to a range that you like to complete the task, Ralph Bustamante said.

"Whether you punch him or you hit him there's no some hesitation," Ralph Bustamante continued. "And this means that there's an opportunity to follow-up. Many people believe they'll only have to hit once and that's enough. For instance, a lot of beginner boxers will strike their opponent and sit back, proud of their accomplishment. On the street there are people who take great satisfaction whenever they hurt somebody."

Of of course, you should not allow yourself to be struck in order to cause an instant of hesitation, Ralph Bustamante said. If it happens do not panic. "One hit is usually not likely to cause you to fall off," he said. "So use it to your advantage. It lets you in so that you can switch the ranges and perform whatever you've been trained in doing."

High Range

"The high range basically runs starting from the shoulders upwards," Ralph Bustamante said. "Street fighters are more likely to strike the neck, chin , and nose regions. Sometimes, they will attempt to break an eardrum when they know exactly what they're doing."

If you're facing an attack of high-range, shift to a lower distance. "If you're in boxing style, you should go to the midsectionarea," he advised. "If you're interested in punching, move to the legs or shins or apply your knees to reach in the middle."

If a person attacks high or low, is it a matter of whether you fight at the middle or low range? "In an on-street fight you should go to the is the target you are able to reach prior to going there," Ralph Bustamante recommended. Like Bruce Lee said, use your weapon of choice to strike the closest goal.

Be aware that it is best to shift to a jeet-kune-do area that the opponent isn't familiar with. Because many boxers and street fighters have had experience with punches to the abdomen it's best to stay clear of that. "If you're comfortable with the way he's doing the way he's dealt with, don't be around," Ralph Bustamante said. "Instead you could hit the shin, step on the foot or your groin."

Middle Range

The middle region includes the ribs, sternum and stomach. "Getting injured in these places hurts and could cause you to be off the road," Ralph Bustamante said.

"If someone tries to hit your in the middle then he must lower his hand," he continued. "Then you can choose to go either high or low. I'm more at ease in the high positionand countering with a hit towards the eyes or nose. Keep in mind to not hit the person directly into the head, and risk breaking your hand."

A large number of fighters, particularly those who were inspired by muay Thai like to kick into their legs, but they'll go for higher strikes when the chance arises, Ralph Bustamante said. Since this type of fighter will likely be protecting his head when he is blasting your mid-range and you might want to focus on his low range.

"You might try taking off his leg that supports him however it could be difficult to hit since you must remove his kicking leg in order in order to reach it," he said. "Or you can block the kick by knee smash or sidestep and hit low."

Low Range

The low range encompasses all targets that are below waist. It is evident that they are the most easily attacked using the legs. "There are occasions that attackers will kick low and you can place his middle by slapping him on your sternum" Ralph Bustamante said. "It'll make him look like a fool."

In the typical street-attack situation you will see your opponent duck his head and attempt to tackle you in the manner of an athlete, Ralph Bustamante said. "Most people are unaware that all they need to do is lift up the knee, and then strike from in a different direction which is where the chest and face are often exposed. This can be a shocking awakening."

Moving back and pushing the attacker's head back is effective, however most people don't think about this, Ralph Bustamante said. "That implies that it requires some additional training. The most straightforward thing to do is to elevate the knee and utilize your survival instinct to defend yourself."

If you're playing the lowest tackle you're likely to sink, Ralph Bustamante said. "If someone is low enough, it means they've prepared themselves. So, it is important be able to fall correctly and then do the follow-up. The force of the fall could be extreme, and can cause knee pain. If he is lower than your knees, it is impossible to be kneeling him as your knees are moving up. If you fall make sure you are ready to apply the kind of bicycle kicks that are used to increase his range to help him get out."

As grapplers constantly remind the world of martial arts that you should be at ease on the ground, Ralph Bustamante said. "It is a must for all martial performers."

Advanced Skills

Once you are proficient at changing your ranges, as mentioned above, would you consider changing your range more than once during an identical fight? For instance, if an attacker is punching you in the face, should you strike into his middle range, and then kick to his low range, and then possibly return to your middle range?

"Confusion is always a good friend," Ralph Bustamante said. "But when something is performing well, it's difficult for you to choose another thing. It's your choice and your feelings in the moment. Your reaction to the attacker will determine what you should do next. In the event that you don't get what you're looking for, you'll need to make changes."

This is where women are able to stand out from males, Ralph Bustamante said. "They aren't trying to be competitive because they know that they aren't able to beat men. They begin to search at the other options which are available. This is the way that men should view it, too."

Exercise Routine & Diet

"Absorb the valuable. Dismiss what isn't." These eminent words are frequently associated with Bruce Lee, and while it's unclear if they actually came from him however, it's clear that they form the basis of his martial art. The legendary and varied combat style Jeet Kune Do, "the method of intercepting the fist" was focused on constructing his attacks around the opponent's attack at a point where anything extraneous could cause him to slow down, with disastrous consequences. In the end, the fighter was extremely unpredictable and entertaining.

39

The flexibility and openness of his approach also determined the way Lee was able to approach his physical training. While the trainers and his fellow students were occupied with territorial disputes and a search for training programs that are universally applicable, Lee was receptive to various practices. Lee absorbed what he needed from bodybuilding, martial arts as well as other types of training. He was dedicated to kettlebells and barbells and also adored his Nautilus style Marcy Circuit Training. He trained his punches and kicks every day at full speed, but he also cycled, ran and rope jumped.

In essence Lee was an all-around athlete. The outcome was an athletic body Joe Weider once described as the most sculpted he'd ever seen. Forty years after Lee's tragic loss, people remain captivated by his unique combination of strength, speed, and elasticity. Just some new pictures of him in his shirtless outfit is enough to merit a feature story.

Naturally, Lee never trained solely to look attractive. His goal was to create an efficient body and appearance was an outcome of his education. Training, as he stated consisted of "the art of showing our body." This is the way he achieved it and what you can do to achieve the same.

Punches: Monday/Wednesday/Friday

Jab-Speed Bag, Foam Pad, Top and Bottom Bag Cross-Foam Pad, Heavy Bag, Top and

Bottom Bag Hook-Heavy Bag, Foam Pad, Top and Bottom Bag Overhand Cross-Pad Heavy Bag

Combinationsof Heavy Bags Top and Bottom Bags, Speed Bags for Platform Workout

* Chest, back, biceps, calves: 5 sets, 15-20 reps, 30

second rest period

• Cardio 5 min warm-up, 12 mins high intensity,

5 minute cool down

Kicks: Tuesday/Thursday/Saturday

Side Kick

Hook Kick

Spin Kick

Front and Rear Thrust

Heel Kick

* Quads, hamstrings shoulders, triceps and shoulders: 5 sets, 15-20 reps 30 seconds intervals of rest

* Exercise: 5 min warm-up, 12 mins high intensity, and 5 minutes cool down

Sample Cutting Diet

"Meal One: 10 scrambled eggs whites. Three servings of of cream of rice, 1 cup oatmeal 3 rice cakes 24oz of water

* Meal 2 6oz skinless grilling poultry breast, 1 cup of grits and 6oz yams. 1 cup of asparagus steamed and 24oz water.

* Meal 3: 6oz tuna, 1 cup brown rice, 1 sliced cucumber, 24oz water

* Meal 4: 6oz perch fillet, 1 cup barley, 6oz baked potato, 1 cup steamed green beans, 24oz water

* Meal 5: 6oz pork tenderloin, 1 cup brown rice, 6oz sweet potato, 1 cup peas, 24oz water

"Mateal 6" includes 10 scrambled eggs whites. 3 servings of cream of rice, one cup of oatmeal and 24oz of water

The Rock Dwayne Johnson Sample Muscle Building Diet

* Meal 1 - 10oz cod, 2 eggs 2 cups oatmeal

* Meal 2 - 8 oz cod, 12 oz sweet potato, 1 cup veggies

* Meal 3: 8 oz chicken 1 cup white rice and 2 cups of vegetables

* Meal 4 - 8 oz cod, 2 cups rice, 1 cup veggies, 1 tbsp fish oil

* Meal 5 - 8 oz steak, 12 oz baked potato, spinach salad

* Meal 6 - 10 oz cod, 2 cups rice, salad

* Meal 7 - 30 grams casein protein, 10 egg-white omelet, 1 cup veggies (onions, peppers, mushrooms), 1 tbsp omega-3 fish oil

Workout for Muscle Building

This is a muscle-building exercise routine utilized by The

Rock, Dwayne Johnson.

* Day 1 Shoulders

"Day 2" - Home

* Day 3 - Legs

* Day 4 - - Arms

* Day 5 Chest

Day 1, Shoulders

* In a seated position Military Press Machine - 3 sets x 21 reps Dumbbell Lateral Raise the super set Dumbbell

Front Raise - 3 sets x 8 reps each

* Rear Delt Cable Raise - 5 sets x 12, 10, 8, 6, 4 reps * Hammer Stength Shrug - 5 sets x 12, 10, 8, 6, 4 reps * Four Way Neck Machine - 4 sets x 12 reps Day 2 - Back

* Large Grip Lat Pull Down 5 sets x 12 10 8 6 4, 4-reps Close Grip Lat Pull Down 5 sets of 12 10 8 4 4, 4 reps * One Arm Seated Row Machine 4 sets x 12 reps. Back Extension 4 sets x 12, 12 12, 12 reps Day 3 : Legs

* Leg Press 4-sets x 25, 20, 18 16, 16. (Last set is a drop the set) *Smith Machine Lunge – 4 sets x 8 reps per leg Lying Leg Curl 4 sets of 12 10, 8, 6, reps

* Standing Calf Raise 6 sets of 16 repetitions (Last set is dropped

set)

Day 4 - - Arms

* Alternating Dumbbell Curl 5 sets of 12 10 8, 6, 4,

Reps

* Preacher Machine Curl - 6 sets of x 12 10 8 6 21 21, 21

Reps (*Last two sets were 21s)

* Cable Tricep Extension 5 sets x 12 10 8, 20, reps * Overhead Cable Extension 4 sets of 12,

10 8, 20, reps Arm reverse Grip Tricep Extension 2 sets of 15 reps

Reps

*21s are 7 upper half part reps. 7 lower partial reps.

Reps and 7 full reps. 7 full.

Day 5 Chest

* Incline Dumbbell Press 5 sets x 12, 10, 8, 6 10 8 6, and 4 reps Dumbbell Bench Press - 5 sets x 12, 8 4 4, 4 reps Cable Crossover - 4 sets each 12 reps

* Pull Ups 4 sets of 15 repetitions (superset using crossings) Abs are practiced every week twice, using a Weighted Swiss ball

crunches. 4 sets of x 25 reps.

JKD Techniques For Grappling And New Directions In Training

Kicking, punchingand grappling, and trapping -- the four facets of combat are included in every discussion of Bruce Lee's jeet-kune-do. With the demise from Dan Inosanto and the late Larry Hartsell, none of Lee's own students have concentrated on the fourth range. Which is ironic considering that grappling is a hot topic nowadays. This exclusive interview with Dan Inosanto, Inosanto discusses the frequently overlooked issue of JKD groundwork,

45

and as it was practiced in Lee's time and also as it is being practiced today.

Many believe Bruce Lee's jeet kune do was just about kick-boxing and trapping but that's not really the entire picture It's not true at all. When sifu Bruce was living, he studied grappling art forms like Chinese chin-na wally Jay's jujitsu, Wally Jay's and Japa-nese Judo, and was trained by Gene LeBell. In Tao from Jeet Kune Do, he clearly demonstrated grappling techniques -throwing, locks and submissions. If you look at the opening sequence of Enter the Dragon where he's grappling Sammo Hung, how does him finish the Ght? Through an submission.Why would you believe the majority of people don't get beyond Lee's kickboxing nunchaku, trapping, and kickboxing? Bruce recognized what was great on camera. Most of his techniques used in his films are focused on striking which is not because he was unable to do other things

, but because he was aware that the particulars of grappling are extremely difficult, if not impossible, for cameras to capture.Just take a look at mixed martial fights. In the beginning, of the Ultimate Fighting Championship, the referees wouldn't get the fighters up again when they were when they were on their feet for the longest time but the fans began booing and the promoters had acknowledge that the watching public wanted to see the action or else the money could go somewhere else. It could be a tiny twitch of the hips, or fighting for grips however, if the viewers aren't able to be able to see it, they won't appreciate the action. If they don't understand the action, they won't be able to appreciate it.The another reason he did not show the same amount of grappling in his films is that it was because it was an

tions...

The field was still relatively new to his knowledge. He had a ton of hours of punch, kick and trap instruction, however his study of grappling arts was at its beginnings. If he wanted to film something, sifu Bruce wanted to excel at it.But the grappling expert was constantly examining the range of ground and even began creating chi sao on the ground. But, in sifu Bruce's lifetime, grappling was more than stand-up game.Was grappling an integral part of the syllabus at the Chinatown school? Sifu Bruce taught submissions and locks on the ground, as well as takedowns, however they were not contestable. That is we practiced them to aid in technical improvement, not as a form of sparring similar to what we practiced when we did kick-boxing. We did not fight one another like we did in kickboxing.What did he did was to work on specific things with students individually during his private lessons. When he gave private lessons, he would not solely focus on what would be the best for each individual and their own JKD -as well as train himself in the process of developing his own abilities in a specific range.One one of the aspects that made him stand out in his abilities was the ability to shift between kicking and punching range , the trapping range and then to the grap-pling range. At the time, all martial artists were able to excel at a particular area. In the event that you kicked, did not punch or wrestle much. In the event that you punched you did not kick or wrestle as much. If you wrestled it was not the same level of proficiency in striking. Sifu Bruce was ahead of his time with the way he trained him and students in order to make them skilled in crossing the gap between ranges.Are there different ranges within the grappling? Of course. The range that is referred to in Tao of Jeet Kune Do as the tie-up area, that is the stand clinch range. It's the same thing that wrestlers now do by the pummeling. They are using an upper collar that they hold. They hold the bi-ceps, triceps, wrists and neck, forearm and so on. These clinch techniques are extremely beneficial to strikers since they enable them to secure their opponent and allow them the time needed to recuperate from a devastating strike or breathe. Grapplers need to master this technique, otherwise they'll not be able to cross the gap and dominate adversaries on the floor. They have strategies like overhooks, underhooks, and two-on-one technique to aid them in achieving the takedown. It's a much more difficult game than playing on the ground, however they're all part of the overall game of grappling.Did Lee teach drills that included ground strikes? No. They were added after his death due to Shooto people such as Yori

Naka-mura who taught them to us in the years 1989-1990. Due to working with Yori I realized the need for groundwork in the first place, and when I began to learn about Brazilian Jiu-Jitsu in conjunction with Renato Magno and the Machado families as well as Renato Magno I definitely realized the need for ground work.I have incorporated a lot the moves that I learned from Shooto and Brazilian Jiu-Jitsu's vale tudo instruction along with the striking, trapping and grab-pling techniques I learned from Sifu Bruce as well as other instructors. While I'm not saying that the way I'm practicing is 100% right, but these are the foundations of our ground game. And we credit the information that comes from where. There are also influences from other systems of grappling -dumog, which was taught to me by Juan LaCoste, Naban, which is the bando py-thon method that was instructed to me by Dr. Maung Gyi, and others.Bando does have a grappling method. It's an interesting history lesson. We often believe that

tions...

There is a reason why something is not mentioned in the time when there isn't exposure to it through the media however this doesn't mean it was not there. Mixed martial arts have been practiced for centuries. Bando for instance, is a kickboxing and weapons sport, as well as wrestling, yet only a few people were aware of the sport prior to. Why is this happening now? Because of the money associated with MMA as opposed to people simply doing it as an ancestral or cultural treasure.Even at those Hawaiian sugar plantations, decades ago, Filipinos were engaged in MMA. They fought with kickboxes and grapples using sticks, and also trained

daggers. Today, we are more aware of the coverage on TV as well as Internet exposure.Many people claim that trapping has its own distinct category and is not the same as grappling. What do you think? Trapping is easier when it's when you're on the ground. The ground eliminates one of the vectors of motion which restricts the opponent's movement and makes him very difficult to find. A skilled shootwrestler or BJJ practitioner is aware of trapping at a higher level however, he isn't required to use the term "trapping." It is possible to refer to it as "clinching" as well as "pinning" and "holding," but all these terms refer to the same thing as trapping. In the example above when someone hooks your arm , or grasps your arm and then strikes you or throws at you, you're trapped. A trap doesn't have to be a pak sao or lap sao or something like that.On the ground, can you employ a variety of percussive or striking techniques?Absolutely. You need to be able to draw into and out of any circumstance requires or what force your opponent offers you. Just like I said, Brazilian jiujitsu is a very effective trapping art. advanced practitioners may hold your arm in a trap and move into a position that gives them more leverage and advantage before attempting to punch or striking your opponent. It is important to understand the trapping technique in Brazilian Jiu-Jitsu, for instance it is about gaining control of a limb, which allows control over the body of your opponent before attempting to submit. While I used to train together with sifu Bruce standing up, he'd get control of two of my legs for a few seconds and strike me three or four times during a trap.Perhaps due to the early UFCs that there was lots of debate about the fact that boxing isn't effective when you're on the floor. However I've heard Ray "Boom Boom" Man-cini could even weave and bob across the floor. Does that sound true. When we were in training I was watching him grab someone from the guard while he was practicing vale tutudo. When the person who was in the guard tried to throw punches at his opponent, Boom Boom bobbed and moved around until he discovered an opening to either use his punches, or a surrender and control. Boom Boom didn't need to learn that. He simply applied his natural instincts as a world-class boxer. It is possible to apply the majority of what can be done standing on the ground, as long as you know the context. The clinch technique he acquired in stand-up boxing serve him effectively on the ground.Some instructors say it is difficult to generate strength when hitting on the ground. Boom Boom Mancini can uppercut your guard and it's going to cause a lot of ruckus. It's not a difficult task to knock out a shot every time. All you need to do is put some shots and you'll be shocked at how much your opponent's skill or level of ability decreases. In the late Carlson Gracie said that the first punch that an black belt gets could transform him into brown belt. Two punches later, the belt becomes an orange belt. Then, after three strikes and three punches, he's operating at the level of a

tions...

The blue belt's technical proficiency. At the age of four, blue belts are in survival mode.A punch could also be an opportunity to set up a different technique such as an attack-by-drawing sequence. A punch can be used to cause irritation, but only to make the opponent raise his arms and, in turn, provide you with the chance to alter your position to gain control, and then make an effective submission.What do you think of the legacy of Lee's grap-pling? My personal opinion would be that sifu Bruce might have believed that it's fine to study other grappling styles, such as shooto and Brazilian Jiu-Jitsu. I believe that if there was information about those systems, he would have studied the systems to find out the aspects that were valuable.These times, we employ certain methods and techniques to teach JKD. When I instruct I always state, "This move came from shoot-wrestling" "This series is from Kali," or "This move was derived from Brazilian Jiu-Jitsu." We keep the integrity of the techniques taught by Bruce sifu, but we don't shut one's eyes from the positive aspects of other systems.I have the rank of senior shooter under the guidance of sensei Yori Nakamura Black belt in Brazilian Jiujitsu under Rigan Machado, and a sixth-level black belt under the Dr. Maung Gyi, but regardless of my accomplishments I am aware that I need to be more efficient and educated. Although I learned grappling from masters like LaCoste, Tenio and Subing the art shooting, BJJ and Erik Paulson's Combat Submission Wrestling re-ned my knowledge of grappling.It's like going to someone's home and you can't just walk through the front door to see everything comes from a single store. There may be a object, such as couch, that comes from one shop as well as an end table that comes from a different retailer. So long as the whole can be seen functionally and visually, no one is making a fuss out of it. This is JKD. You don't need to be a fan of all information that comes from one source or rely on one source for all the information you require. The things we have and the tools we do as individuals must be tailored to our preferences and capabilities. Rigan Machado once told methat "You aren't a fan of the whole system of BJJ instead, you should embrace the aspects that work for you in BJJ.

You don't change to BJJ but rather take from the jujitsu that is adapted to you."Some people will argue, "Don't call that 'JKD grappling'" since what we're teaching may be just 40% of the techniques Sifu Bruce taught, however whatever worked in his case may not be the best for you. JKD grappling is the result of experimentation, research, creation and improvement in order to develop the system of grappling that is suited to the person. It is a shared, experimentation, and learning process in my academy and is in constant evolution.Street grappling is changing. In the 1960s, no one knew how to kick as a street ghter today. In the present, thanks to the media's exposure, even the non-trained attacker is more comfortable with grappling. Conict, war fighting, combat, ghtingwhatever you choose to define it -- there is always a change. If your combative technologies and tactics don't change and evolve, you could be in danger of extinction. The core of JKD is still alive, however it's the human body, and its application of it have advanced to become aware of all aspects of combat.

Manual Blocking Made Simple

What does this mean for warbands or manual blockage?

It is possible to have a 25 percent possibility that you'll be able to block the swing, If you are able to block the swing randomly in one direction. If your weapon is unable to move, you'll have a 33% of a chance, and if the weapon is limited to two attack directions, you have 50 percent. It's also possible to use the spear-like weapon that is that is shielded, in which all you have to do is to block downwards.

This chance of blocking can be greatly increased through this method. Gun Kata method.

Based on the position of the enemy, as well as your location You can calculate that:

* In the majority of situations, your enemy will employ"short swing" in most situations "short swing" or, he'll swing from the side that is closer to you.

* If he is on the stairs or in a building etc., the likelihood of him taking an upward swing is increased.

* When he's facing you directly the likelihood of an explosive thrust is increased.

If you are unsure you should put your block to the left. Statistics show that this will be the best way to stop hits.

For those who don't know you can block lancers by making an upward block (won't cause couching to stop).

Firearms Instruction for Close-Quarter Combat

You might have to poke them in the eye

Law enforcement is a job that is in close contact with the public in general. To fulfill their duties officers of the police must always be within a double-arm's distance of their fellow citizens which I refer to as The Hole. In this region, police officers have the greatest risk and there's no way to stay out of close proximity with people and suspects. Consider the outrage that could be caused by officers sitting back 30-40 feet and shouting at a person, "Sir! Take your identification off and bring it back to me. I do not want to be close enough to you, for security motives!" As for suspects they can't be properly taken your suspects in custody safe way without touching them and putting them in handcuffs.

For many years the most risky moment for any officer comes when the initial handcuffs are put on the wrist of a suspect.

Therefore, it shouldn't come as a shock to learn that the vast majority of shoot-related incidents that involve police officers take place at distances under 10 inches. There are most of them happening within The Hole. You'd think that the majority of instruction in firearms would be conducted at the same distances, but it's not the reality. The truth is that training for close quarter shooting can be challenging and possibly hazardous, and a lot of agencies simply don't practice it.

In the last five or six years I've had a lot of thought about how law enforcement can prepare for the most extreme close-quarter shooting scenarios. I've looked into what's happening in this regard across the nation and have spoken with officers who've had to deal with similar circumstances. No matter how good or not I'm also the product of my own experience and I'm not able to help but look at the current methods of teaching to the ones I've been through in my own personal experience. After more than three decades in police work, much of it in roles like

SWAT and narcotics operations, and night-watch patrols I've accumulated a decent number of first-hand experience that I can draw from which I believe is lacking in the researchers and instructors currently developing theories of training and the latest the latest trends.

In this regard and with the possibility of pointing some the current doctrines of training in the eyes I've determined that the best method to prepare for shooting close quarters is to

Combat...

Be simple and don't overload the process because experience has proven that keeping things simple works the best. The idea of imagining a method for every scenario is attractive, yet we are aware that this is not feasible. In light of the fact that the vast majority of police officers train/practice only when they're scheduled to undergo in-service training, it is sensible to stick to the SIG rule: Simple is good.

Simple Combat Techniques

First, you have to be aware of is that the firearm is not the best solution for every situation, even if it is necessary to use deadly force. If your surroundings are The Hole, introducing a gun could lead to the person who is armed with it employing to harm you. My personal opinion based on my personal experience is that when you are confronted with a the distance of two arms, you should use easy-to-use (but very efficient) hand-to-hand combat techniques including knee elbow, palm-heel head-butt and forearm strikes. Unfortunately, these tactics are being replaced by more complex techniques for controlling subjects like the use of wristlocks and pressure points grappling, and arm-bar takedowns. This is a shame, as to break free and allow the room for a firearm to be used, you have to strike with force on soft areas of the body.

Additionally, keep in mind these three things:

* You are not able to draw a holstered gun against a weapon already drawn.

* Action always wins over reaction, unless you perform something

something to deter the attacker

* If a firearm or knife is present, that weapon should be the primary target in the attack and not on an person.

If you can get your weapon perhaps you could be able to add your sidearm to the fray. However, this only applies if that the officer has good gun holstering skills. Many police officers on the streets cannot pull their firearm from their threat level 3, 4 or 2 security holsters in under five seconds, making the possibility of bringing it into play in such a scenario a risk. Retention of the weapon is essential but not at the cost of being able to use your weapon swiftly when required.

Be Prepared to Do Harm When It's

In my early days of work I was behind an ambulance along with the largest female patient who was being transported from an institution to a mental health center. In the course of transport the "lady" was upset and, shockingly was able to free herself from her restraints, and attacked the ambulance driver. His reaction was to jump out of the ambulance, and the driver actually speeded up to make it to the hospital. As I was being tossed in the rear in the ambulance. The patient reached to my holster Smith and Wesson Model 66 revolver. The battle was in full swing. I tried the different pressure points that I had been told could turn a suspect in combat to Jell-O. But none one worked. I was amazed by the strength that this woman had when she was throwing me around. She finally grasped my weapon and refused to allow me to let go. I knew it was just a matter of time until she took control of

Combat...

it. I solved the issue by performing a super-secret, Ninjalike, spec-ops move that is only known to a handful of people around the globe I poked her right in the eye with a gun. She released the gun and grabbed her face. the battle was finished.

In my early years I realized that one must be in a position to breathe and see to be able to perform any physical activity. Interrupting or affecting the ability of your opponent to perform. This strategy worked for me against playground bullies. However do not think this is as simple as it sounds . Your adversary's neck and face tend to remain in continuous movement. Strikes or claw-like strokes that hit the neck and face are easy to master and require no training However, they do require dedication. You have to be prepared to cause injury to your opponent - an act that many individuals, even when faced by death or injury are unable to perform. Be aware that you must take part in the rescue of your self.

There are those who say that face smashes and forearm strikes on the neck aren't effective in actual fights, but you'll need to prove it to me. I've tried this strategy at least three times (besides my small ambulance ride) during my time in the sport and it was successful every time. Keep in mind that I never received any training to perform the maneuver, other than being able to straight-arm when playing football. Each of the three incidents involved an attempt to disarm me and each time, the method allowed me to have an opportunity and the space needed to draw my arm and manage the situation. If there was a weapon in the mix I would have tried to gain some distance (non-firearm) or disengage the weapon prior to initiating an attack. Can a face-rake be sure to work? It's not a guarantee - there's no guarantees in a fight , however, I'm willing out on a limb to say that if you make strong contact with your eyes or nose to draw your opponent's interest.

Live-Fire & Simulation Training

When you have a good understanding of basic strike techniques I suggest that you engage in both live-fire as well as simulation practice (Airsoft and SIMUNITIONS) to understand the particulars of close-quarter shooting. This type of training will not be in the form of drills at the square-range and requires you to step out of your comfortable zone and engage (actually be physically violent) with fellow officers trying to release their sidearms from their firearm's holster. It's quite an exercise that must be experienced in order to be comprehended. Following dry exercises, it's time for intense close-quarter live-fire drills. The live-fire drills I like to use in training require threedimensional targets, such as the TAC-MAN or full-size mannequin from Law Enforcement Targets These targets let you hit the target with a realistic way, and can also move from between sides in a human-like manner. It's more difficult to hit a target when it's moving around. Also, having the shooter to shoot the gun in their eyes is an educational experience on its own.

Incorporate the forward and lateral movements necessary to be able to withdraw from an actual combat, and you'll get the most realistic live-fire exercises. Start slow at the beginning and be cautious that serious injuries could occur during these drills when you're not focused on the task at hand.

Combat...

doing. But, the reward you receive from this effort is worth the effort.

Dry-Fire Concepts

Do not just do the exercises -- improve your techniques! Start by setting a target for the entire session. Select one specific area that you want to improve in your training session. This could include improving your grip on the gun drawing, stance and reloads as well as trigger manipulation, relaxation as you perform at higher speed as well as movement when drawing various places and more. Next, take about two to three minutes to imagine the result you would like to have from beginning to end. Create a film of what the performance should be as and how it should feel. Make sure you are clear about the way you'd like to go about it.

Work on achieving a perfect two-handed grip, drawing and connecting securely with the firearm prior to fully extending. Feel the pressure of your fingers, and the wrists becoming stiffer and making sure the trigger finger is relaxed and relaxed. Practice shooting the trigger in the same direction from beginning to end without squeeze any other fingers in the gun's hand. You could also try out techniques for tactical movements such as reloads, high-speed draws and any of these. If you're simply playing around and not working to improve your skills You aren't taking as much benefit from every session as you can.

* Work at different speed and using different starting locations, targets, and dry fire firing courses. Make use of both block training where you perform the same skill for a set amount of repetitions, and varied practice that allows you to do different variations each time you perform it. It could be as simple as changing the place your hands or gun begin from, the size of your target as well as different ranges for the target, conditions that are light as well as incorporating movement of the body as you perform the skill and so on. This improves the internalization of the

technique and results in an improved performer.

Start with 25 % of total speed, then gradually work up to 50 percent, 75 percent, then 90 to 95 percentage of the speed you believe to be your highest speed at which you can perform the technique effectively 10 times in one row. You can gradually increase your speed without compromising safety until the technique begins to unravel. You're in the 100-105 percent range or what I call"the RED ZONE. This is the area of improvement.

This is extremely important do not slow down every when mistakes are made, unless it's a safety concern. Find a way to fix the mistake by focusing on the place where the error originates and then focus on performing that task at the same time you made the error. If you don't begin doing this, you'll never become much faster or more proficient and you will be at an unattainable level of skill what you could be. If you can't correct the error, return to a slower speed, and be aware of the way you're doing it to ensure you are doing it correctly , then work your way back towards the RED ZONE.

After you've completed the technique until a maximum of 200 repetitions, take a quick break.

Now, you can put your focus in the arena of performance or shoot-out! It is essential to aim for the right emotional state and keep it throughout dry firing. If you don't, then you don't have the right mental and emotional conditioning and you are just going through the movements on a physical level.

Combat...

Learn to master the art of gunfight speed that is between 90 and 95 percent of your top speed, for 25 to 100 repetitions, with the intention of performing in a gunfight, qualifying or anywhere you would like to be successful.

Each session should be brief, but focused. Focus on your mind must remain sharp while you remain aware of what you're doing as you do it. For the majority of people, 15-30 minutes work well.

Sample Firing Grip Exercises

Here's an example of what I'd be doing when working with a student to improve their grip for firing to get them ready for a greater standard of proficiency. Start with these dry-fire exercisesThey require the highest focus to execute them correctly. You'll find yourself doing all sorts of things you didn't realize what you're doing. You'll need shooting equipment and an electronic timer (ideally one that has an option for partime) should you have one. Be aware that live ammunition is not permitted inside the dry firing zone.

Exercise 1: Use a timer when you have it and set a par of 4 seconds

* Goal: Increase the awareness of leverage, friction and the control that exists between the hand and the firearm

* Instructions Draw the weapon slowly, achieving the perfect two-handed grip when you reach the area of the. Make sure you don't pull the trigger. You should feel your hands securely in contact with the gun. Maintain the same grip tension each time you complete the exercise. Repeat this exercise for 25 times.

Exercise #2 - Time of 4 seconds

Goal: Manipulating your trigger whilst maintaining the proper hold tension to the firearm. Maintain constant pressure when controlling the trigger.

* Instruction Repeat the exercise, however, now press the trigger with your hands remain in the gun. Perform 25 repetitions. Make sure you are aware of keeping your link to your gun by using your grip for shooting.

3. Exercise 3: Create a timers for the par time of 4 seconds.

* Goal: Different training drill that helps you to learn to achieve an ideal grip from various hand starting places.

* Method: Similar to for exercise 1 however, start by using a different position for your hands every time. It is possible to do hands facing forward and hands holding objects behind, hands in the back, hands mimicking using a rifle, etc. Try 25 times, using a different starting position every time. Find a grip that is perfect each time.

Exercise #4 The par time should be set for 3 seconds, then slowly reduce to 2 seconds each 10 repetitions until you've completed 50 reps.

* Goal: Reach greater awareness and control of your shooting grip by firing and drawing

while gradually increasing your speed between 50 to 75 percent top speed.

* Instruction: Repetition the exercises 1 and 3 at the highest speed trying to achieve the perfect grip every time.

Exercise #5: Determine the time limit for between 1 and 1.5 seconds.

* Goal: Growing in speed outside from your comfortable zone towards the Red Zone, strive to get a perfect grip

Combat...

link between the gun and the hand, both prior to and when using the trigger.

* Instruction 3. Repeat the exercise at a higher speed for between 50 and 100 repetitions.

Exercise #6

* Objective: To perform the skill at gunfight pace and incorporating the proper mental concentration and conditioning.

* Instructions Set the timer to the speed that corresponds to 90 - 95 percent your Red Zone speed. Do 25 important, repeated repetitions while imagining yourself in a real gunfight, or some other important occasion.

A lot of repetitions? No, not really. You can complete this entire course in between 25 and 30 minutes.

These are just a handful of the dry fire exercises that I have designed to teach my pupils. Your only limitation is your imagination.

This series should be completed three times per week, every day for at least four weeks. There will be immediate results from your live-fire training because of an increased awareness of your grip when you shoot.

Chapter 5: Kicks Spinning

Let's review the most well-known ones to begin with.

Make sure you're stretching and warmed up prior to starting in order to decrease the chance of injuries that can occur to this type of exercise.

-

It is the Spinning Back Kick

Absolutely, it is among the most effective techniques in martial arts.

It is best used for frontal attack and performs equally well close-range as it does from the distance.

It's an excellent offensive and defensive method that stops the opponent in their lines.

However, despite its name it is true that if you actually spin with this kick , you are more likely to do it wrong since the footwork to spin for the back kick is actually more twisting than spinning.

To make it easier to understand I'll demonstrate the technique in the right lead (left leg ahead) and kick using your right (rear) foot.

If you can, as you're attempting to perfect this move, you should locate an even line on the floor, which you can use as a reference.

It's not necessary, but it will prevent errors that are made at the start of the process.

-

The Part that is striking

You can use either the heel of your foot, pulling the toes back.

The edge or side of the foot. It is also called"the foot blade..

Test both options and determine which one suits you.

Personally, I prefer the heel to the sword of my foot.

The attitude

Because of the nature of kicks the most effective position to execute this is a stance that is sideways.

A side stance is when you place on both heels in the same line in order that your toes face toward the side.

Set your kicking foot at the back, and then place your back fist on the chin (rear Guard).

When you're in a side stance, you must ensure that you're not exposing your sides of your body. Hence, your arm in front (lead guard) is utilized to cover this part on your back (as as shown in the image above).

Do not raise the fist of your lead guard further back than the knot on the belt you wear for martial arts, or the buckle of your regular belt, or your belly button (if you're not wearing belts).

A further move back can pull the arm in the direction of the back and exposes the back of the body (which you might not observe).

It can also be used for further travel if you want to take it on to fight.

In simple terms, Your dominant hand will be the strongest one. It is the one that strikes to the back as well and can be (generally) employed as a punch of power (knockout type) punch because it will generate more power and force as it moves. While your weaker hand is usually located at the front, and thus closer to your opponent, and is thus used to increase speed and knock down an opponent, and allowing you to throw the big knockout blow.

The same principle is applicable to the kicks.

The breakdown

Ideally, to ensure that this kick will take place in the initial stages of your development , you should be near to the opponent or the target.

I'd try to get a touch distance and from your stance on the side you can just reach the target with your fingers that are on your lead hand.

When you are more skilled using this kick, you are able to increase or decrease the distance.

1. Begin facing your goal (or adversary) with your back as illustrated (below).

2. Turn your feet around to ensure that your entire body is facing the opposite direction. Your goal is directly behind you. Make sure that as you do the twist to make sure you don't block your right leg by using that leg on the other side. Look at the next image below to learn what I'm talking about.

3. Your head should be turned to the side so you can glance at your right shoulder to check that the target isn't moved.

4. The right leg should be dragged backwards along the flooring in a straight line.

This easy technique is sure to ensure that your kick is hit dead center and prevents the spin-off effects that occur when body mechanics are not correct.

5. When the leg is passing through your body, raise it upwards and then attack the target using your foot or heel sword

Tips & Hints

The most common desire is to let the guard down in kicks.

It is a terrible way to start and is difficult to overcome once the foundations are laid, so try to avoid this at all cost.

Be sure to pay attention to the position of your foot so that you can ensure that the kick performs at its fullest.

The supporting leg must be set away from the goal in this moment to ensure the body mechanics are correct.

Once the kick is hit, you have the option to land the leg on the front of the body for a potential second attack or return to the original position.

-

The Kick in the Reverse Round

There are a variety of terms for the kick, and every one of them will vary based on the type of art you are studying or the country that you reside in.

No matter what you decide to refer to it, the fundamentals that make up the kick without doubt be the same, and is the reason why the kick is found in a variety of other martial arts because of its versatility and effectiveness.

The striking portion of this kick is the same for hooking kicks (see "Martial Arts for Beginners PT1 - Fundamental Kicks')

It is best done in a side-on posture.

It's also intended to attack the back of an opponent. It is due to the movement in the kick it is an extremely effective technique.

It can be utilized in the for high, middle or low section. It can therefore be used by any person with a degree of its flexibility.

The most striking part

Before we get into the reverse round kick , it is helpful to know the part of our foot we will use to kick with.

Simply put you can find two major components of the foot you can utilize.

1. Heel of the shoeusually used to destroy.

2. A flat, or ball for the feettypically used for sparring.

The position

Because of the nature of kicks The most effective stance to use is the natural side-on posture.

Front facing view

Side facing view

A quick note on stances

In my prior ebook, you've probably come to realize that for almost all standard spinning kicks, the best and most effective stance to begin is to take a side-sit when performing them by yourself especially when you first begin to learn these kicks.

The reason why a side stance is so more straightforward to start with is that you're already halfway to where you want to be.

If you begin in an aft (facing) position, you need to change to the side (facing) position and then keep going with the kick.

The common sense would dictate that a side-sit eliminates the bulk of (unnecessary) move.

It is true that... it is true that you are able to perform a spinning kick from any stance. It's just that you'll need to do a more work. Which is great however my thoughts are first, let's try to make it as simple as we can you to grasp and, of course, make it the easiest way to do each spin.

Also, if you need to work harder, it's likely to take longer (and although we might only be talking about milliseconds, that could be enough for an experienced opponent to defend or fight back) and thus you run the risk of communicating what you're going to accomplish.

I'm at a point now (having been doing this for over 30 years) in which I'm able to know what my opponent is going to be doing well before they even start by their posture or how they move, and how they carry their own bodies.

In addition, there are the fact that there are a few steps you don't need and the complex nature of spinning kicks (and we'll not even get into it the fact that they're much slower than static, basic style kicks) and you're not going to have a chance that a spinning kick could be involved in fight.

As we move through these spin kicks, I will show you the kick with different postures.

If I am fighting or sparring I like the idea of fighting (or spar) with an angle as it is what works best for me. So often I am able to throw a kick that spins with a more angle position.

-

The breakdown

We'll begin by focusing on the leading foot side kick.

1. Make sure you face your opponent with your stance of fighting.

2. Turn your feet around so that your body faces the opposite direction and your target is right behind you.

3. When you begin to spin and spin, make use of the energy generated by this spin to lift your kicking foot off the ground.

4. Maintain the leg straight and let it be completely circular in its line.

5. Also, turn your upper and hips around to add some force to the kick while you kick the leg that you are kicking through until it reaches its goal.

Tips and Hints

After you've executed the kick, you should try to land with your kick leg exactly where it was to return you to the original lead.

It is also possible that this can be helpful should you choose to perform another technique, in addition to helping you in maintaining your balance.

Maintain your leg straight throughout the kick, and remain as upright as you can.

Keep the guard in place throughout , and avoid the usual error that many people make when they kick this way and let the back hand fall off and leave the face exposed.

A Spinning Hook Kick

The kick is an improvement of the earlier one (the opposite round kick) and was created to create an elongated circular kick without the limitations of a straight leg kick.

When the leg stays straight and straight, the rate of spin becomes decreased, which gives you a better chance of counter-attack.

In addition, the tightness of the leg may make the kick a bit difficult to perform.

This kick permits the body to move at a more rapid rate because the leg is in a coiled position until the last second and adds additional energy to the method by the whipping motion towards the final.

-

The most striking aspect

Like the previous kick it is made to target the side of the body using the same strike tools.

1. It is the heel part of the feetusually used for destruction.

2. A flat, or ball for the feetusually used to spar.

-

The breakdown

In the beginning, we'll concentrate on the hooking kick that leads leg.

1. From your preferred fighting posture.

2. Your feet should be turned in such a way that your body is in the opposite direction and your goal is in front of you. Make sure you look at your right shoulder to your attention at this point.

3. When you begin to feel the energy of the rotation then lift your rear foot off the floor , and keep your knee up.

4. You can then whip your upper body and hips to extend the leg.

5. When the kick reaches its spot, you can hook the leg by whipping it in order to boost the energy.

6. Then continue to the back.

7. and back into your stance.

Tips and Hints

After you've executed the kick, you should try to land your foot back to the direction it started from in order to return you to your original lead.

This will assist you if you want to try a different technique as well as help you maintain your balance.

Maintain your body as straight as you can during the primary portions of this kick. You should also make sure to keep your guard in place to avoid the mistake that people make , which is to drop the rear hand , leaving the face exposed.

Note the location of the foot supporting it in the primary place of contact.

The most frequent mistake that individuals make in the large most kicks (basic or advanced) is that they do not comprehend how the supporting leg operates.

To get the body in the right place for the kick to get the maximum impact, ensure that the heel of your support foot is in line with the target. This will help open the hips, and aid in balancing.

-

This is the Spinning Round Kick

This particular kick spins ideal for covering distances and is equally effective when directed towards the body or towards the head.

The device is intended to hit on the sides of your body by a circular motion.

Like most spinning kicks, the more you spin, the more effective the kick is. to speed up the rate of attack, try it either from an angular position with proper footwork, or a side stance.

-

The most striking part

Before we get into the actual kick, we need to recognize which foot part we strike with.

Simply put it is that there are two primary components of the foot can be used to kick the round with a spinning motion.

1. The foot's ball is usually utilized for destruction.

2. The instep, which is generally employed when sparring.

-

The breakdown

This kick may be done in many different ways.

Because of the complexity of spinning kicks, let's take a look at what I believe to be the simplest version to use here.

1. Take on your opponent in the position you prefer.

For the demonstration I'm on the Left leading position (so my right leg will be ahead). Keep in mind that at this point of your training , you have the option to opt for a side-on-stance or an angle posture. Based on the next movement it doesn't matter what stance you choose to start with since you'll end up in the exact same position.

2. Take a step behind your front foot by extending your rear leg, so that the rear leg falls on top of your body, while your body is facing in exactly in the same direction. This technique is also referred to as 'cross stepping' since you're stepping across the rear

of your front leg as well as making a "cross by crossing your legs.

3. Then, begin unwinding the upper body (clockwise) to prepare in preparation for kick. Make sure you spin your head around as fast as you can to ensure you don't lose track of your opponent. Be aware that when you turn, you alter how you lead (your left leg now is ahead) therefore, you must switch your posture also.

4. Continue to rotate as you raise (chamber) the knee in the same way you normally do to prepare the kick. From here, it's the matter of deciding the direction you'll kick based on the goal that you have at your disposal.

5. When the spin is winding out and the kicking leg returns towards the front, use the momentum that you've created at this point to hit the kick with the maximum force.

-

Tips and Hints

The more you move your rear leg when it crosses step (at the beginning in the process) and the further forward you'll go, which means this kick is a great option extremely effectively to cover a distance and also create a lot of speed thanks to the winding movement at the beginning.

The kick is described in detail to make it easier of understanding, the quicker you spin , the more efficient.

Be aware of the fact that turning back to the opponent even for a moment is always risky. So make sure you fully commit to this strike immediately you begin.

A Spinning Outside Crescent Kick

As I wrote in my previous publication (Martial arts for beginners The Kicking Series Pt 1 - Basic Kicks) the crescent kicks were initially intended for close range combat and the spinners aren't an the only exception to this.

They are also distinctive because they are the only spin kicks that the body is held straight throughout. It's because of this that they work particularly well when used in close proximity.

The only issue you might encounter in this type of kick is that in order to create the power needed for its effectiveness the body has to completely rotate, which temporarily makes it vulnerable to attack.

So there is a tendency not to observe spinning crescent kicks to the same extent as the spinning hooking kick, for instance, since fighters are getting better in their ability to recognize them and consequently, better able to fight them or avoid them.

-

The most striking aspect

The most striking feature of this particular model is the external part of the footspecifically the outside of the heel.

The breakdown

To better comprehend the body movements required to spin, you have to imagine that you have the pole that runs vertically across the center of your physique (from head to the toe) and down to the ground.

This will assist you maintain the proper body posture throughout the complete move of this kick.

1. From your stance of fighting.

2. Turn your body clockwise and remain the body as straight as it can. Take note that for a short time you will not be able to clearly see the subject (or you opponent in this instance) so you should make this technique very quick.

3. Turn your head to look at your shoulder to the opposite side and concentrate on the target you want to hit as you continue to reverse the turn.

4. Transfer your body's balance and weight onto your lead (left) leg. This serves as pivot point.

5. When your right shoulder is brought in line with the goal begin to lift your kicking leg off of the floor. If you do it correctly it will be a matter of speed and momentum of the first turn will cause the leg to turn.

6. The only thing you have to do is maintain your balance, continue the spin , and reach the goal.

-

Tips and Hints

If you do it properly If you do it correctly, the momentum and speed of the first spin will result in the leg whirling through, so concentrate on the spin instead of trying to push the leg round.

To make it easier to get the hang of this, simply hold a stopwatch with the string with arms length and then spin it around fast. The speed of the rotation will (if performed correctly) result in the watch to raise. This is what you should be doing by using this kick.

You might notice that your supporting leg flexes slightly as you kick it may also rise on the foot's ball. This is completely normal when you perform this kind of kick as the leg that supports you will act as a shock absorber to assist in balancing and rotate.

It is also possible that your leg you kick is likely to bend at the start of the kick. This is also perfectly normal if you extend your leg fully by the point of contact. If you do it correctly it will be straight by itself when the spin has reached its the maximum speed.

Don't lift the leg that you kick off the ground until the very last second. This will accelerate the kick and improve your balance.

-

It's the Spinning In Crescent Kick

The concept behind this kick is the same as the "Spinning Outside Crescent Kick" but using the inside of the foot for striking during this time, and then adding an additional step in order to make up for the shift in strike tool.

Spinning Inside Crescent Kick Spinning Inside Crescent Kick relies on the spin's momentum to power the kick and at same time to cover distance, consequently, the spin used for this particular method is vital.

-

The most striking aspect

The most striking feature of this model lies on the inner side of your footspecifically the inside of the heel.

The breakdown

I'm going to demonstrate this in an angled stance using an angled left lead (left leg ahead) but you might prefer it easier to use a side stance in the beginning since you'll need to include an additional movement to allow this kick to be effective and a side stance may aid in this.

Check out how you do.

You can also apply the same "pole through the body" principle for this kick to help get the right motion.

1. From your stance in a fight.

2. Your body is twisted backwards (clockwise).

3. Your your rear foot (right leg) is turned around and ends up on the front.

4. When you land, utilize your landing leg (the one you just landed on -- the right) for a pivot point and continue to spin until your left leg rises (chambers) up to prepare to kick.

5. When the kick is at the center line Straighten to straighten the (left) knee to be sure that it is hitting to its fullest potential.

6. Allow the momentum that the kick generates to carry through, landing your leg naturally before returning to your posture.

Tips & Hints

When you begin your spinning, ensure that you glance over your shoulder , allowing you to concentrate on the object, as shown in the second picture above.

It is also possible that once the kick has landed in the rear, your supporting leg could be bending slightly. This is also a normal element of this kick since the back leg functions as a shock absorber in the same manner as it was for the earlier kick.

If it doesn't alter you balance or balance, this shouldn't affect your kick.

The speed is the most important aspect of this kick, so even though the physics of it have been broken down significantly, the faster you spin, the better chances of it getting to the ground.

However... this is an extended drawn out kick. So when you practice it, I'd recommend setting it up using something that is basic and then when you've got your opponent on the backfoot (moving forward) then attempt this kick in order to pursue them and attack them all simultaneously.

This is the Spinning Axe Kick

A spinning kick usually utilized to strike the opponent's front in a downward direction or, if executed properly, because of the speed of the kick it is also able to take on the opponent at an angle (as illustrated in the "Martial Arts for BeginnersThe Kicking Series -- Pt 1' eBook). The Kicking Series -- Pt 1. The Essential Kicks' eBook).

It is typically used to make attacks with high sections (unless you are bent by your adversary) so the ability to move is crucial in this type of attack.

The fundamentals behind the spinning kick of the axe is the same the static version . It is most effective to take on the side that is blind to an opponent.

This is an ideal strategy to use against a competitor who prefers the opposite lead to yours or that changes leads during the battle, since you do not have to switch to them to fight the blind part of them.

The most striking aspect

The striking point in this case will be the sole of the shoe -usually used to destroy.

The feet's flattypically used to spar

The breakdown

1. From your preferred position

2. Your feet should be turned in a clockwise direction until your entire body is now facing the opposite direction. Your goal is in front of you. Make sure you look over your shoulder for a focus at this place.

3. When you begin to feel the energy of the rotation then lift your rear foot off the floor , keeping your knee up to help in the movement of the kick.

4. Extend the leg while you continue to spin.

5. As you turn towards your opponent, you should drive the kick straight downwards in a vertical direction.

Tips and Hints

Because of the difficulty the kick is a bit awkward, knowing the technique required to bring the leg upwards and hold it while driving it down is essential.

For speed For speed, bend your knee while you spin, and only straighten it once you have started your turn, facing the adversary.

The kick must be set at a point that it can be able to pass over the shoulder of your opponent while you spin. If not, it's most likely to land on the shoulder, or even miss completely when you're too far from.

When you have reached the center line then stop the spin, and then drive the forward straight down.

Another option is to alter the hips' angle slightly so that your kick is now at an angle, with your focus being on the side of your face.

You'll need to learn the kick slowly to get it mastered, however be cautious with the spinning axe kick since it requires an enormous quantity of timing, speed, and practice to be able to work in a realistic setting.

If you can get this you'll be amazed!

Chapter 6: Gun Sau Drills

Important Note

The most common reason people are frustrated by martial arts is because they become too competitive. GUN SAU is built on the abilities of balance, sensitivity and flow. If you start to get intense before you've learned these techniques, you'll tighten up and push the opponent, which can turn the game into a wrestling contest or you'll attempt to beat their pace by going faster than they will be.

The best method to improve control, sensitivity, and balance is to practice slowly and put aside any competition until you have mastered. If you have MA education with WingChun, Ki Chuan Do, Tai Chi, escrima or something else, you'll be able to learn Gun Sau faster because it is similar to flow drills in these styles, like Chi Sau, hubud-lubud and many more. If you don't have any long-term MA training, then go really slow and simple to play it like dancing or playing until you are able to master it. The idea is to have enjoyable! !

STATIC GUN SAU

In this exercise, you will take a an upright, wide stance and cross your forearms, but you are unable to shift your foot. You can change how you balance your feet with straightening them and bend your knees. This exercise is a good way to test shifting the weight of your body (which is the source of power) as well as to develop basic arm strength.

One-Step GUN SAU

You can now do one step at any time during the exercise however, you must take a ten second break before making another step.

TWO-STEP GUN SAU

Similar to the drill with ONE STEP but you'll be able to take two STPEs

PIVOT/STEP GUN SAU

A different variation of the drill ONE STEP however this time you must remain with the same foot (right or left) on the floor. You are able to pivot your foot, but you cannot walk along with it. The other foot can move around however much you'd like.

One Hand Gun SAU

This can be done using the STATIC one-step, two-STPE drills and the PIVOT/STEP. In this drill , you will only use the gun arm to traps, parries and so on.

SLOW MOTION GUN SA

This can be done from every drill. It is recommended to begin slow regardless. If you do move, it is best to slow down.

Gun Sau Drills 71

Too fast too quickly or become too competitive, you won't develop a good techniques. If you go too fast or get too competitive, you will not develop good.

KILL ME! GUN SAU

Tghis may sound odd, however it is extremely effective. The majority of people become too competitive and find themselves wondering why they aren't getting good at what they do. This is because they are running before they are able to walk. Make use of this KILL ME! drill when you're going too fast, trying too hard, or simply not having fun anymore. You can use the drill to say Kill Me! anytime, and you can let your body open to be shot. This is the most effective way to remain loose, and develop your ability by doing this. I guarantee it! !

BLINDFOLD GUN SAU

Blindfolds can help you focus on sensitivity and the ability to position.

SAU DISARM/RETENTION GUN

In this practice, you're not shooting the other player, but you try to get their gun and prevent them from disarming yourself. It is also possible to do different variations where one person is unarmed while another is arming.

FREESTYLE GUN SAU

It is the best and most sophisticated drill. Simply move around freely and use all of your abilities to shoot and trap, disarm, and so on.

14

Gunfight Training

To prepare yourself for a real-life shooting scenario on a busy street, you have to extend your range beyond the shooting limit of the range.

Training firing angles:

In August 2012 officers were able to confront a homicide suspect that had shot an individual outside of the Empire State Building. As officer approached him and he pulled out his gun and the officers reacted with a shot into the person. In the course of that incident, nine more were injured in the aftermath of the fire.

you can see the officers reacting as they have probably been trained -- they stand, draw their weapons and fire. I'd like to suggest that the majority of police officers that read this are taught the same way.

73

In this particular scenario, there are many residents who are walking or driving by.

In the nearby buildings, there are thousands of others. The total number of shots were fired from officers. These rounds struck towards the suspect's level with the ground, at around chest level, which is the angle that is most likely to hit any person walking or driving through.

Variable Angles of Fire

As I stated earlier, the officers may have responded as they were taught to. In such situations, you might want to think about changing the angle you shoot from by lowering your shooting to knee or even prone to decrease the risk of hitting someone with an unintentional miss or a bullet that is too deep.

In hindsight, it appears that the huge planter featured in the video could have given the chance to go down low and then angle the shot upwards -- the angle which would have taken the bullet's path over those who were watching.

The old saying states, "What goes up must be brought down." This instance, it is important to choose the one that is less dangerous. A bullet that goes up into a building , or the office window is less likely to cause serious injury as compared to a similar shot on the street.

One of the major issues with our education is that we are constrained by our facilities for training. The majority of ranges do not allow sharply angled shots either to the left or right. All shots that aren't parallel to the floor will end in hitting the ceiling, the floor or crossing the berm at the outdoor range. Every range you go to requires that you ensure that your shots are placed in the safe backstop that is approved by the range -in turn we accidentally reinforce the notion that straight shots are safe while shots that are angled can be dangerous.

We all know that when you've never been trained to do something, don't think you'll be able to perform it with a lot of pressure during a fight and even in shooting.

5 Key Factors to Consider

There's an appropriate time and location when the strategy of shooting an angle shot that is steep is worth considering. Here are some suggestions to be prepared for such situations:

1. Practice. The range at which you shoot may not allow live shooting at these angles. Instead, use an instructional pistol, or even better an FX marking pistol, Airsoft or even a BB gun. Paper targets are fine however you should use a 3D target is more effective and live targets are most effective if you adhere to the correct safety and training procedures for equipment -- based on what you want to shoot.

2. The angle of the shot changes and the angle of the shot is also altered. A shot that could hit the heart straight in may go over the top in a shot taken from a lower angle. 3. The aim can change. If you've taken the position that is lower in order to ensure that your shot doesn't hit the person you are shooting with

or bystanders who are nearby, you might be able to shoot higher to the chest or the head to ensure that the trajectory of your shot is clear of any innocent people within the range.

4. Know the anatomy. In the course, you should look at an anatomy chart and sketch the appropriate targets and bullet path from various angles and heights to ensure you have the greatest chance of successful bullet placement.

5. Try working on angles. Try standing, crouching kneeling, squatting and everything else in between to achieve the angle you require. You can practice close to as well as at a distance since you'll never know the exact distance that the gunfight will take place.

Get ready for the real world in 360 degrees. It is important to practice range shooting however, the range isn't the real world and you're limited to the directions and angles you are able to shoot according to the layout of the range. Create your practice "real" by creating scenarios which require you to fire angled and mentally practicing the steps you'd have to follow to create an effective as well as safe(r) shooting, paired by red or blue gun training with a partner in training.

Make sure you are firing an FX airsoft or pistol at your live, moving, breathing threat , if you have access to this type of weapon.

The test of competition and self-esteem:

There's a time when you might want toor have to -determine what you're made up of in situations where there are serious consequences to failing. Although we are able to evaluate our own performance in a variety of ways, I've noticed that the majority of "testing" scenarios aren't able to reveal what you could accomplish under pressure. Additionally, many training situations are too cold and controlled to allow the proper, "full-on" testing.

To me, a real evaluation of performance has five parts:

1.) The scoring process is objective and as it can be

2.) A reward that is of significance to the person who is being examined

3.) Perceived failure's consequences are proportional with rewards

4.) A worthy challenge

5.) A worthy opponent(s)

One of the best method I've found to measure my own abilities is to participate. In 33 years of competition you'd expect me to have a good grasp of what I can accomplish. However, this year brought some surprise for me.

It is the USPSA Handgun Nationals

The USPSA Handgun Nationals was held in St. George (Utah) and consisted by two National Championships held back to back. This Limited Match was initially held as a separate competition to aid in the creation of the teams from around the world which would compete for America United States at the World Championships next year. In the next event, an Open and Limited 10 Nationals. Open as well as the Limited 10 Nationals was held the following day.

Shooting competitively -- particularly at world-class competitions is among the best ways to get to know your gear, yourself and your mental state and also your physical and mental preparedness. It can do things to you that are virtually impossible to duplicate in a classroom. Smaller events or competitions in-house aren't as stressful weight of major events (but they're an excellent way to begin).

The year that I joined, I was part of my "super squad" that included all the top shooters. Since then, I've been on this team several times before but haven't been there for several years due to the fact that I was instructing my pro-team shooters, and shooting together in their squads.

I entered this game hoping to do good. I had set my targets and they mattered a lot to me. But, over the course of three days, I'm not sure I was able to settle down enough to shoot as well as I'm confident I can. There were some great shooters on our squad: Rob Leatham, Nils Jonasson Dave Sevigny, Bob Vogel and Members of the Army Marksmanship Unit, and many other outstanding shooters.

Everyone was still making mistakes as if we'd just learned to shoot.

It was a challenging set of matches , with a lot of hard shots and numerous opportunities to make mistakes that were utterly embarrassing. However, it wasn't until after I got back home that I realized I had been examined -- actually checked! In a way that I hadn't been for the past few years.

I wasn't prepared for the competition that I witnessed in this group. Instead of remaining focus and calm I was constantly trying to push the pace and making a lot of mistakes. It wasn't just me! Everybody in the group was doing similar things every now and then.

I was letting my subconscious mind take over shooting, making sure of things I would normally perform automatically, and slowing my speed. I noticed that I was missing steel targets and had to reconnect them as it was my intention to knock them down. I was too fast in my the move from one position to another and shooting poorly instead of focussing on hitting properly. The pressure I placed on myself to do my best was not recognized until I was unable to make amends.

While I performed pretty well in both of the matches but I was not able to do what I'd like to -and I wouldn't give it up for any thing!

I found my limits. Physically, mentally emotional, and physically. figured out my strengths and areas where I could use improvement.

I realized that my glasses prescriptionthat I believed to work adequately in the past did not meet the requirements of the task and the rate at which I needed to take in the information. I discovered that I was emotionally and mentally overwhelmed and needed to shoot against this degree in competition more frequently basis in order to adjust to it. I realized that I had to make a few minor adjustments to the gun to be able to shoot more effectively.

Although success can boost confidence, it can also encourage one to work more.

instead of fretting about acquiring the "training scar" I view the failure to be an opportunity evaluate my mistakes and weaknesses with a critical eye and begin fixing them in a systematic manner. Instead of blaming myself or rationalizing my mistakes I can see the areas I can improve on. I then can create an instructional plan to tackle the trouble areas.

Test of Self-Sufficiency Test of Self

Self-testing will test your determination and ability. The test will assess your strength as well as your discipline and judgement. It will test your ability to be present moment and function in the subconscious mind when your conscious mind is trying to control and control the situation.

While competitive shooting might not be your thing I would suggest all to find something you are able to participate in that is significant to you. It takes the determination to step out and put your ego on the line, try your hand at it and discover what you're made of.

Accepting these tests and the judgement of your own self when you truly consider them to be a serious matter you will soon find yourself seeking to improve and making steps to improve. If you consistently strive to improve your performance, you'll be better equipped to deal the challenges that life can throw at you.

That, my dear fellows, is the reason we have to test ourselves.

You've learned how to dearm a gun several thousand times, and now you're at the point of skill that you are able to remove anything other than a shotgun out of the hands of your trainer.

However, a handgun disarm involves more than swift fingers and a willing partner. If you want your handgun to be prepared for the eventual "gun at your back" encounter the timing of your disarm must be spot on.

Although handgun disarming techniques are few in close combat DVD's nowadays the most important aspect is frequently left out...

...and it's probably the most crucial step in your technique of disarming.

This is about the correct timing of your dearming handgun!

The thing is, your attacker is already pumped up when he's got his gun pointed at you. most times, the head is focused on the weapon and you as his "target". In this mindset any impulsive move by your side could trigger a quick release of the trigger whether on purpose or in reaction to your sudden move.

Sure , it is helpful being quick to move your body away from the line of firing. To successfully complete the handgun's disarm, you must be sure to time your movements so that his brain is not focussed at the trigger.

In order to accomplish this, the brain of your attacker is to be separated from the trigger finger. In the realm of psychology, this is known as"break state" or "break state" which is a brief psychological "hiccup" that occurs when the brain is focused.

To aid you in your attempt to disarm There are two frequent times that your attacker is in a breakstate during a hostage incident...

...but only one gives you the chance to disarm the gunman and change the rules.

Below are some options...and the winner is:

The Handgun is Disarmed "Break state" #1: If You Receive Orders from the Gun Owner

When an attacker gives instructions to you to perform something your brain is temporarily focused on communicating the directions.

In that moment it is very unlikely that he will be likely to pull the trigger since the brain has to first engage to shoot. It could take only just a fraction of one second, but during disarming a firearm the smallest fraction of a second could make the difference between life or death!

However, this break-state isn't the best way to take down a person with an assault weapon.

Why?

Many people, particularly the smug thug who is armed with a firearm, will give directions using their hands. Therefore, even if he's the state of break when he's directing for you to go from one place to the next it could be that he's using his gun to direct you towards the direction he's directing you to go.

If you make your disarming attempt while he's giving you instructions It's highly likely that the gun is moving and you're than likely to fail to reach your intended target once you try to disarm the gun.

But, there is an alternative...

Gun Disarm "Break state" #2: After He's Given You Instructions

If your attacker has given you an order or requested that you move your brain is more focused on ensuring that you're following his instructions. This is a more effective break state since the movement you make is something you are the only one who can control it. your brain must determine whether or not it's the one he requested you to do or if he has to give you more instructions.

It is the best moment to move in and get the gun!

Here's why...

1. Because your adversary isn't providing direction, but is rather focused on your personal move and is less likely to see the gun moving.

A well-balanced handgun provides you with a an unchanging "target" to focus on during your move to disarm. It also improves your chances of getting it right.

2. If you're being asked to move, the person asking you to do so is expecting your body to be moving. So, your quick and light move is more likely surprise him because the movement you performed was something you were asked to perform initially.

3. This gives you the ability to speak to your adversaries. When you're speaking to the other person, the focus of his brain is again diverted away from the trigger and the disarm is harder to spot. It's even more likely to happen if you're moving while conversing simultaneously for example, asking "You are referring to moving over here?"

In your training for disarming with your handgun do not just practice the actual disarm movement. Practice with realistic scenarios that resemble hostages as well as create mental break states for your adversary to master the whole handgun disarm process.

Think about these scenarios:

Scenario No. 1

It's late in the night. You're walking to the vehicle in the parking structure. Your mind is distracted and you're not aware of the surroundings. In a flash the man walks from the shadows. There is no way to glimpse his features, but see the semi-automatic gun in his palm. It is just a few feet away and is pointing towards your chest.

"Give me the keys to your car immediately!" he orders.

In shock and scared with the sound of the shot, dive into your pocket and take out your keys.

"Give the items my attention!" he commands, and you do as he commands.

"Back up. Go back!" Again, you comply with the instructions.

The gunman takes the keys, then gets into the car, and then drives off.

Scenario No. 2

It's dark. You're walking towards your vehicle in an parking structure that is lit by a couple of dim lights scattered too away. Your mind is busy, and you're not conscious of the surroundings as you should be. Unaware the man walks from the shadows. There is no way to look at his visage, however you see the semi-automatic gun in his palm. It is only a few feet from you and is pointing towards your chest.

"Give me the keys to your car today!" he orders.

In shock and scared at the sight of the firearm, you reach into your pockets and pull out your keys.

"Give the items my attention!" he commands, and you comply.

"Back up. Return!" Again, you follow the instructions.

The gunman seizes the keys, but then turns away, shouting "Now go into the trunk!"

The first scenario offers an obvious argument to comply to the demands of a gunman. A gun is a major danger to your safety. If you are able to ensure your security by providing him with what he wants then do it. Your vehicle, your wallet, and even your jewelry are useless. The moment you return back home to your family is the most important thing in your life. The events described in scenario No. 1 are reenacted in the street of America every single day. Unfortunately, the same is true for the scenarios described in 1 and 2. 2. You can co-operate with an attacker who is armed and provide him with all the things he demands and yet be in danger of death. The most frightening aspect is you could not be aware of the danger you're in until it's too to late. This unsettling, simple fact is the primary reason to include realistic gun defenses within your defensive tactic arsenal.

Krav   maga
[http://www.blackbeltmag.com/category/
krav-maga/], the official hand-to-hand combat system of the Israeli Defense Forces, includes some of the most practical and effective techniques in existence -- techniques that are relied on by soldiers and police officers who face armed threats day in and

day out. The techniques taught by krav maga for gun protection can help you develop strategies that can be used in a variety of scenarios. This decreases the number of tactics you have to master and remember, resulting in a less time-consuming training and quicker use under pressure. For instance, krav Maga employs the same method in the event that a firearm is put anyplace in front of you regardless of whether it touches your body or not. The same method using very small modifications to body defense applies even when the firearm is pointed towards your forehead or under your chin, or on the sides or back of your neck. The krav maga gun's techniques use four principles as the basis for their operation:

Counterattack

Disarm

In most cases, these four concepts intersect. For example controlling the weapon and counter-attacking are often done simultaneously. In order to be able to employ a gun defense to the extreme it is essential to comprehend and implement the four principals.

15

It's the Kata In Gun Kata

As a teacher about Kata applications, as well as a author of articles and books on bunkai, I'm frequently asked about "the proper application" for various Kata moves. It's true that there is no one correct method for any move! Master Itsou was a master who had a major impact on the way Kata is practiced today was once quoted as saying "There are a variety of movements that are part of the art of karate. While you train, you should attempt to comprehend the goal of the move and how it can be applied. It is important to consider all possible meanings and implications of the movement. Each move could have a variety of possibilities." I think that it is vital that the person disengages from

87

Each person has their own distinct understanding and expression of kata application. It is recommended to actively learn about the katas instead of just practicing them, and strive to create efficient solutions from your personal experience. There is no correct or incorrect methods, just those which work and those that do not! In this article, I'll give you a few guidelines for katabunkai that will assist you in extracting useful techniques from the katas yourself.

1. All katas are intended to stop the fight and end it there and. Any technique that could leave your opponent with the ability to fight on is not correct. A good example is the patterns that are usually considered to be multiple blocks without a follow-up. It would be very dangerous by blocking the strikes of your opponent and left in a fight, then why would you want to use kata to do this? The "blocks" themselves have to be executed in a manner to disarm the attacker. Keep in mind that kata applications were intentionally concealed. simply because a move is described as a block doesn't necessarily mean that it was designed to be utilized in that way.

2. All aspects of a workout are crucial. Hands should not be put on hips, or wound up prior to blocking as an preparation for the next method. Each movement is important and a proper application should be able to take all aspects of the exercise into account. If the hand goes towards the side prior to returning to the inward direction, each part of the motion have a function, not just the part that

is inward. Particularly, the use for the use of the hikite (pulling hand) should be taken into consideration. In Gichin Funakoshi's 1925 work"Rentan Goshin Jutsu Karate In the book, there is a small paragraph that is devoted to the use of the hikite. He writes "Here is the significance of the hikite, also known as a pulling hand is to grasp the hand of the attacker and then pull it back while twisting it as tight as you can so that the body is forced into leading against the opposing." It is apparent that the purpose behind the hikite is controlling the opponent's limbs so that they are unable to balance. Make sure you take this into consideration when you study bunkai. Hands should never be placed by the hips to prepare for next moves.

3. Every kata movement is specifically designed to be used in combat. It is crucial to realize that every move in the Katas were designed to be used in actual combat. This includes closing and opening salutations. While certain moves can increase the strength of a person or improve their balance, this is not their main purpose. They are designed to disarm an attacker in combat. In his book of 1974"The Heart of Karate-do' Shigeru Egami wrote, "Despite the lack of

understanding, one shouldn't believe that the moves have no significance or significance. I recommend performing the movements and then thinking about them and then interpreting the meaning in your own way by focusing your the mind and heart. This is called "practice." When you are analyzing your own kata, make aware that each move is intended to combat and try to comprehend the purpose behind it.

4. The angles from when the techniques are being performed are vital. There is no turning back to meet another opponent. The majority of fights don't start; they are typically preceded by a type of heated argument. A statement like "What is it that **** is it you're watching?" or, "Give me your money!" are common examples. A fool wouldn't look at their attacker before striking. The majority of kata strategies are developed to tackle the opponent directly in front of you. The primary reason the kata technique is performed in a certain angle is that they inform the student that they have to be in that position with respect to their opponent to allow the technique to be effective or when they move in that direction, the shift of their body

weight can aid in the execution of the technique.

5. Stances are an integral part of the methods. They are not assumed simply to be attractive or are used to strengthen legs or enhance balance. They are regarded as stances because they incorporate your body weight into the move or help in balancing the opponent. Examine the position and its weight distribution and the shift in weight of the body and the way in which the stance was interpreted. Consider what methods that the change in body weight can help and then you'll take a step closer to uncovering the hidden meaning of the motion.

6. Real fights are messy affairs, and the manner in which the fight is conducted will be a reflection of this. When we perform a kata, we are practicing the "ideal motion. This is relatively simple to master against the thin air, but is completely against another human being that is determined to do harm to you. When performing the kata's methods, the primary concern is the effectiveness of the move rather than retaining the perfect form. A graceful move when done within the kata is rough around the edges when performed in

an aggressive scenario. The aspect of the technique should not be an issue. The only way to judge can be determined by whether the method affected the opponent.

7. The possibility of the attack is to be assessed. Kata techniques mainly tackle the threat of an attacker that isn't trained. Karate is a tradition of civil society and therefore its techniques were not intended to be used on the battlefield against professional fighters. The legendary Choki Motobu once said "The techniques used in Kata were not designed to be applied against professional fighters in an arena or on the battlefield. They were most efficient against someone with no clue about the strategy applied to combat their aggressive actions." Techniques of kata are more likely to serve as alternatives to techniques such as lapel grabs, hooks and head-butts rather than defenses against combinations that are more advanced. Also, it is worth noting that the majority of fights are within close range, so one might expect the vast majority of kata tactics to be suited for use at this distance. Protection against long range strikes like lunging style punches and long range kicks could be considered, but they are much less likely to happen in actual fights

and consequently they will be the smallest percentage of kata techniques.

8. Strikes should be delivered to weak points. There is no doubt that techniques that are delivered to the body's weak spots will be more effective than those that aren't. It is important to be as precise as you can with respect to the locations struck when you study bunkai. It's not enough to claim that a blow has been delivered to the skull's side and not to go to the temple as the resultant effects could differ dramatically. But, it is important to be aware that the exact placement of strikes during an all-out fight isn't as straightforward as some claim.

9. Kata techniques do not depend on the unpredictable response of the opponent, but it is important to recognize predictable responses. It is not uncommon to find applications that rely on the opponent's performance of certain actions, e.g. "it is at this point that the opponent responds by an attack that is back-fist." It is not a reason to believe that the opponent shouldn't respond that way, so this kind of tactic is not recommended. Certain responses are predictable, however they are usually

considered in the context of kata. A person who has received a blow to the testicles is most likely to bend at the waist. Any subsequent movements must acknowledge the same and similar actions that are involuntary.

10. There are many useful applications that can be used for any motion. If your applications are different from those you've been taught or demonstrated this does not necessarily suggest that there is something wrong in the application. If they are effective and conform to the guidelines laid out within this post, they should be considered right.

11 Attempt to grasp the principles on which techniques are built. The important issue is understanding "why" that the methods are effective. It is important to move beyond basic memorizing of techniques and try to comprehend the basic principles on which the katas are built. The principles are more important than the techniques. They can be used in many different ways, however techniques are highly specific , and therefore restricted. The goal is to be an agile and flexible fighter. Try to understand all the fundamentals and how to combat in

accordance to these principles. Although initially this understanding may be at an intellectual level it is important to incorporate these concepts into your unconscious (this is the purpose of kata). In this way, your body will naturally respond in line with these principles, making the karateka very formidable. Through focusing on the basic principles and various ways they can be used the kata is an unending source of martial wisdom and it is easy to understand why masters of the past stated that it takes longer than one lifetime to fully comprehend the fundamentals of a single kata.

12. All applications should be usable in actual scenarios. When you look at the applications consider the following questions: Can this method be used under severe stress? Can it be used in a simple manner or do you need to have an advanced level of skill? Does it have the ability to defeat an uncooperative , possibly physically stronger opponent? Can the technique be used in a real-world setting or am I choosing the first app I found that seemed to match the Kata? Does the technique work against untrained violent attacks or specific karate techniques? Kata applications must be relatively easy to use.

They were created in this in that way. If the idea you come up with isn't feasible, then you should stop and try with a new idea. For every kata move, there are many applications that can be used that you can explore.

Utilize the tips included in the book stay on the right path when learning Juu Kune Do. If you study and practice enough, you'll be able to effectively comprehend and freely communicate Juu-Kue Do in a manner that is uniquely yours.

Chapter 7: Knife Fighting Techniques

Many prefer carrying knives to defend themselves. Like any other weapon, in order to be effective in self-defense it is essential to have the knife in your possession, readily accessible and usable in the conditions. The knife must be at hand and accessible whenever you're at work, in church or at a birthday celebration and so on. You should be able to use the knife even with a heavy jacket or gloves. Also, be capable of holding the knife in hands that are cold or wet.

In a fight, it doesn't how skilled you are or the level of skill that your adversary has, as long as that opponent is armed with a knife, you'll get cut! Therefore, be ready to get cut

127

and not allow a cut to impede your determination to prevail.

It is said that "proximity hinders the ability" that a skilled person can die in combat through mistake. Self-defense is usually in close proximity where an attacker is not likely to stand in the in the back and fight. Therefore, if you'd like to use the knife to defend yourself it is important to be aware of how to use it in close proximity.

Knife

Every knife type can be deadly in fights, but certain kinds are as harmful to the person using them as they are for the attacker. For instance, the cheap folding knives with a the weak lock on the blade which allows the blade to be closed to your fingers. The most important things to consider when selecting a knife for fighting are:

* A fixed blade is more durable than the folding blade. Double edge blade is superior to one edge blade because both sides can cut.

* The point must not be sharply tapered as to easily break off.

* A slightly oval handles are better than a round one therefore you can feeling which way the edges are facing.

The handle should not become slippery after wet. It should not also be or too soft during hot weather or too firm when cold.

The handle should be larger than the width of your hand, so that the butt could be used to strike. Certain knives have a steel pommel that is attached to the butt for more effective striking. If the handle is too large it could snag clothing or be pulled by the attacker.

A blade that has a shiny finish is frightening, whereas the blade that has a matte finish is easier to conceal. * It should include a guard to shield your hands from the blade of your opponent. Guards that are angled upwards help to trap the blade of an opponent and helps you to hold.

Grip

When using a knife you need to hold it. A proper grip essential when making use of the knife, but observing the grip of the attacker could provide a clue to the ability level of the person who is attacking. There are four ways for gripping knives. As with all fighting techniques each has its own advantages and drawbacks.

* Fencer's Grip. This grip is where the knife's handle is held securely between the forefinger and thumb, while the rest of the fingers are wrap over the handles, similar as how the fencer grips foil. Single edge knives are held with the edges facing downwards while a double edge knife is gripped with edges facing up. Blade is pointed towards the person who is attacking. While this grip might be appropriate for knives with smaller handles, it's not suitable for knives with grips

that are large. The grip allows wrists be able to rotate the knife in multiple directions, allowing maximum reaching for the knife and also presents the weapon in a an aggressive way. But, the grip isn't very secure. If your hand is hit with the fencer's grip the knife could fall off your grip of the blade. The thumb could be injured if the thumb slips into the blade or the knife is pushed backwards. This is the grip employed to "flashy" combatants.

* Ice-pick Grip. This grip has the knife handle is gripped in a fist with the blade pointed downwards like you hold an icepick when you are using it to break ice. Single edge knives are placed with an edge facing forward and double edge knives are gripped with an edge facing forward. This grip allows for deep blade penetration through the body, thick coats or any other clothing that is protective However, when you raise the knife to make an upward strike and telegraphing your intent, you signal and expose your chest and make it difficult for your adversary to see the weapon. The grip doesn't allow the ability to parry or thrust, and it is simple to stop any downward thrust. This grip is used by many beginners. The Reverse Grip. In this grip it is held upside-

down with the blade facing downward and forward alongside the wrist. Single edge knives are gripped with edge facing forward while a double edge knife is gripped with an edge facing forward. It is said that this grasp "hides" knives however, it limits the access and techniques. Because thrusts are mostly reversed, you need to be near to the person who is attacking. This is the grip utilized by numerous knife fighters who view knives fights in films and believe they are experts.

The knife fighting technique of pakal utilizes using the grip in reverse. pakal, in the Visayan dialect spoken in the Philippines refers to cutting. Like claws of an animal the movements of pakal are made to grab and tear flesh apart and not to push away. A majority of knife fighters have their edges facing towards the opponent, which means that the person who is attacking needs to fight against the edge to reach them. They make use of knives to stop attackers from getting close. Although most pakal thrusts are backward-facing however, forward thrusts can also be utilized. Because the blade is facing backwards this means that the range of forward thrusts and range of penetration is restricted. In pakal it is the thrust that is the main attack motion. cutting, shearing or tearing is considered to be secondary. If you force an attacker away, he is likely to strike once more. This continuous disengagement and reengagement provides many chances for things to be wrong. When you strike forward the attacker is likely to move back to prevent or reduce the force of the strike, then return to the strike for a second attack. If the attacker is able to pull back, he or will be able to move into the force of the strike. If the attacker doesn't pull back the strike will move forward towards the attacking. When someone is cut they tend to move away fast, so when a cut is cut while preparing to make a backward thrust it can cause the victim to back-flip to the thrust.

In a fight with a knife in pakal it is not necessary to fight with your opponent and engage in a long duel, you employ deceit as well as feints, speed aggression, and a variety of strategies to stop the fight in the shortest time possible. Because pakal involves lots of ripping and thrusting, using a blade with a shorter length with an opposite grip is the most effective weapon.

You could push against the edge of any blade using greater force than you press against it. Attackers aren't always naked. They wear clothes and, depending on the conditions and season it is possible to have many layers of clothing or even heavy clothes. It's hard to cut through skin with the layers of security. When a thrust is made forward, the person who defends is typically moving backwards away from the attack , which means it's difficult to cut the clothes even with a big blade. But, if a smaller blade is pulled towards the body it is much easier to penetrate clothing as the clothing is backed by the more solid layer of body.

Due to the clothing and movement of combat, the shorter knife is less likely of being caught or snagged. When you thrust it only a tiny portion that is the size of a long blade can penetrate, which means it's difficult to gain enough leverage over the handle to manage the knife. A blade that is short may be able to go through to the hilt however this provides the user with immense leverage to pull and tearing. If a larger blade is pushed too deep or hits bones, it can get stuck and be difficult to get out of. The additional leverage of smaller blades aids in its removal from the same.

* Hammer Grip. This is the most preferred grip for experts. In this type of grip the knife's handle is held in the same way you would grip with a Hammer. The blade is pointed upwards. A single edge is held in a forward-facing position. A Double edge knives are held using the edge facing towards the forward. The wrist stays flexible, but it can be locked at any time. By using this grip, knives are less likely to be thrown out of your hand and allows the hand to strike or deliver butt-end knife attacks. The grip offers powerful penetration and strength, so the blade can easily cut through clothing that is heavy. Additionally it is less likely of injuries to the thumb and the knife can be used for cutting or slashing and, in particular, thrusting techniques.

Stance

Keep your normal position of fighting with your knife at the top of your hand. "Hide" between the blade and let it be the only thing your opponent can see. Keep your free hand near the midsection to guard crucial zones. In the Philippines, known as Escrima the free hand serves to protect the body and is sacrificed if needed. The creed reads "You might scratch my hand but I'll kill you!" The free hand could be used to parry, kick or make a fake blow throw objects, disorient the opponent, aid in balance on rough terrain, or to grab the blade of an opponent. It could also be used to entrap the hand of an opponent while attempting to draw weapons.

Targets

Like fighting with your hands in empty hand to take out your opponent as quickly as is possible you need to strike the ideal areas. However, this doesn't mean that you must always hit vital areas. The majority of opponents will defend their main areas which makes them difficult to strike. Because getting the first blood is the potential to be a huge psychological advantage and the more you can hit your opponent, the better, regardless of the place you strike. The primary target is the hand that holds the weapon. By deactivating the hand holding the weapon and neutralizing the weapon, you can eliminate the weapon.

If you do not frequently train in knife-fighting methods, the best choice is to engage in the same way as you train normally, but only that you'll be carrying an extra knife in your hand to increase the arsenal. Utilize the hand that is leading exactly as you would would if you had no knife. Make use of knives to stop the hook, jab or uppercut. If the opponent has knives, you must be aware of the place it is.

Contact fighters are accustomed to being struck. In many cases, they do not attempt to defend themselves because they are aware that they could accept the blow and counter with a stronger strike that they have created. If the opponent has knives and a knife, blocking isn't an alternative. Point fighters, particularly the ippon (one point) fighters, are defeated in the event that their opponent lands a single attack on them, therefore they are taught to avoid or block all attacks. In theory, a point fighter has a higher chances than a contact fighter of surviving a knife strike (when they are not skilled combatant with knives).

A very deadly weapon that is used for Filipino combatants is cutting off the sciatic nerve at the back of the thigh of an opponent at the point where nerve is inserted into the bone of pelvis. If the nerve is cut the leg will cease to function.

The femoral artery that runs along the side part of the leg makes also a excellent goal. If it's cut, the patient is likely to die rapidly. One Punch One Punch, One Kill

The phrase is commonly used in various forms of martial arts, however it is not often used actually. When it comes to firearms they refer to "one shot the one shot" or "one-shot stops" in which an attacker is stopped , or killed with a single shot. Even with firearms the odds are not that high. In some cases, attackers can shoot several times and keep at it, even though slowing dying. Can one-shot stoppers be made using knives? There are three kinds of one-shot stop:

A physiological stop is during the time the central nervous system is cut off (such as when a bullet hits the brain) or where the thoracic or heart aorta is immediately and irreparably damaged.

Psychological stops occur when a person believes that they are supposed to behave in a specific way in response to an injury. A surrender stop is when a person believes that any more hostilities will result in more pain or the death of someone, so the person surrenders.

When it comes to self-defense, the most important focus is not on killing an attacker but preventing an attacker's ability to continue to attack. A stab or cut could result in a surrender or psychological stop. But even a single stab at the heart might not immediately kill or stop the attacker. To be fatal , it must happen quickly. the wound must be at the heart of an vein or artery, or either

*The blood cannot form clots or

*The pressure of surrounding tissues must not stop the flow blood or

*direct pressure isn't applied to stop blood flow. If none of these conditions happen, it could take some time before the patient is bleeding out (exsanguination). Most of the time it will take the transection (complete cutting) of the thoracic aorta in order to cause sufficient hemorrhage to cause unconsciousness between 4 and five minutes. For a 70kg average. (155 pounds) male, the cardiac output is approximately 5.5 1 l. (1.4 gall.) per minute. His blood volume is approximately 60 milliliters. per kg. (0.92 fl. oz. per lb.) equivalent to 4200ml. (1.1 gal.). If we assume that his cardiac output will double

when under stress, Aortic blood flow could reach 11.25 milliliters (~2.8 Gallons) in a minute. If a wound completely ruptured the thoracic Aorta, it will take approximately 4.6 seconds for the patient to lose 20 percent of the blood volume. This calculation does not take into account the oxygen within the blood vessels already inside the brain, which will keep the brain in good condition for longer. The fact is that hemorrhage can be cumulative and, as such, in time, several minor cuts could result in more blood loss than one big cut. Therefore, in order to ensure that someone is quickly stopped by bleeding large veins and arteries have to be cut. even then, it could require a couple of seconds or minutes before the patient becomes incapacitated.

In light of this, regarding bleeding, knife fighters recommend focusing knives on the parts of the body which allow violent movements to continue. They attempt to stop the attacker by targeting muscles, tendons etc. which control arm and grip movement. Like hemorrhage, structural damage can be cumulative, and, just like hemorrhage, it can require a number of cuts before significant damage occurs. The attackers don't sit in the middle of your carving them. They're trying to take you down, which means you don't have much time to play around.

As we have discussed in the previous paragraph, each of the three kinds of one-shot stops are difficult to attain with knives. If you mix muscle and blood cuts together, and the discomfort they cause, you could be able to quickly stopping the attacker.

Knife Defence

An unarmed defense against a weapon is extremely dangerous. Only fight to avoid fatal injury or death to yourself or other people. If your opponent is carrying an axe or a knife, even if you are carrying one, do not fight or leave whenever you can. If you have to engage in a fight, you can employ deadly force because your are the one who has a deadly weapon and is determined to attack you. If you're carrying an axe and your opponent doesn't, use the knife with caution, because you now possess a deadly weapon that could make you legally or civilly responsible for its use, even if the attacker continues to strike.

* If the situation requires it, follow the instructions you are toldto do, including offering up your valuables.

* If you are asked to raise your hands. It's easier to initiate a move when your hands are raised. They are outside of the view of your attacker and you don't appear at them with a threatening look.

• Distract the attacker's attention from your intention by speaking (pleading or crying.). Try to start your defense or attack during between a statement or sentence.

Concentrate on the grip of the knife. Some might think the carry of a concealed gun can protect them from a knife-wielding attacker. The results of tests have demonstrated that a knife-wielding attacker who is less than 21 feet away would be in a position to cut the distance and slice the throat of an inexperienced shooter before they is able to draw and fire each time.

9 781774 858677